TIMELESS MAKEUP

P9-AFY-320
3/13

Rae Morris
TIMELESS MAKEUP

PHOTOGRAPHY BY JASON CAPOBIANCO

ARENA
ALLEN&UNWIN

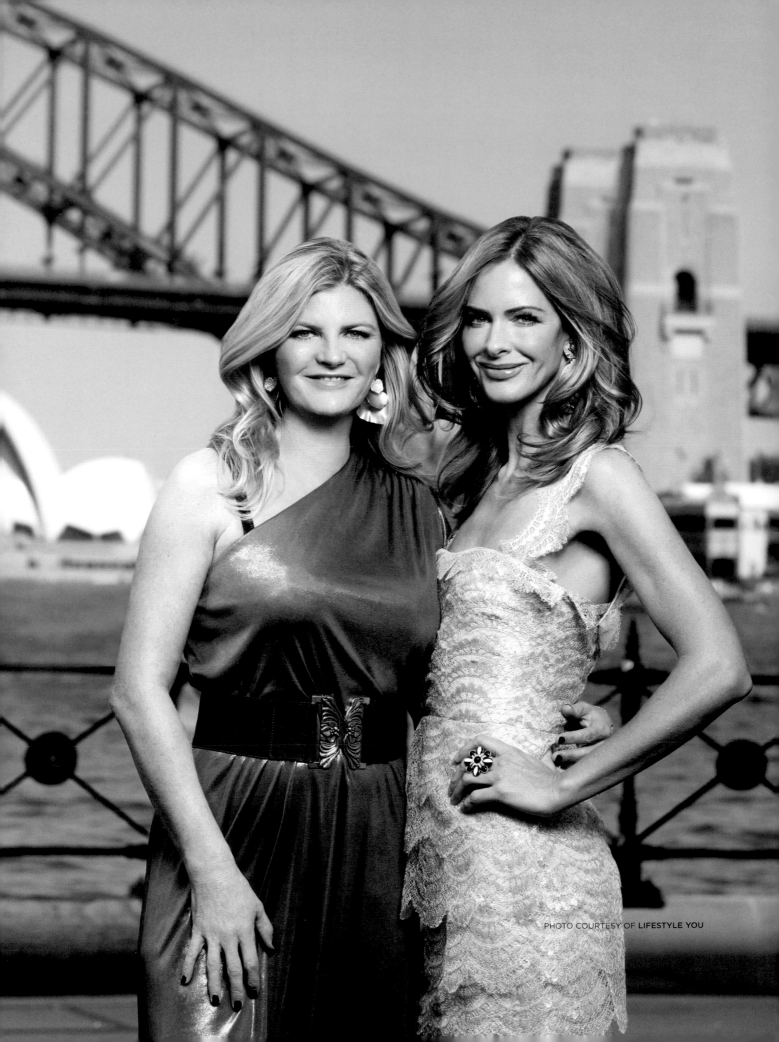

PHOTO COURTESY OF LIFESTYLE YOU

Foreword

Susannah and I worked with Rae Morris on our Makeover Mission Australia early in 2011. We hit hair and makeup straight off a twenty-two hour flight from the UK. I took one look at my face in the mirror as we arrived and thought, 'God help the woman who has to make this look OK.'

Then we met Rae—chirpy, obsessive, generous of heart and mind, and a true professional. We could not have been in better hands. Two hours later, looking like a million dollars, Susannah and I were out on Sydney Harbour, racing around in a speedboat doing the show's intro...until a big wave took it all off and we had to start over.

We spent a month with Rae and by the end of it we were begging her to join us in Israel, our next Makeover destination.

Our only criticism is that she lives on the other side of the world and we get to work with her less.

Trinny Woodall

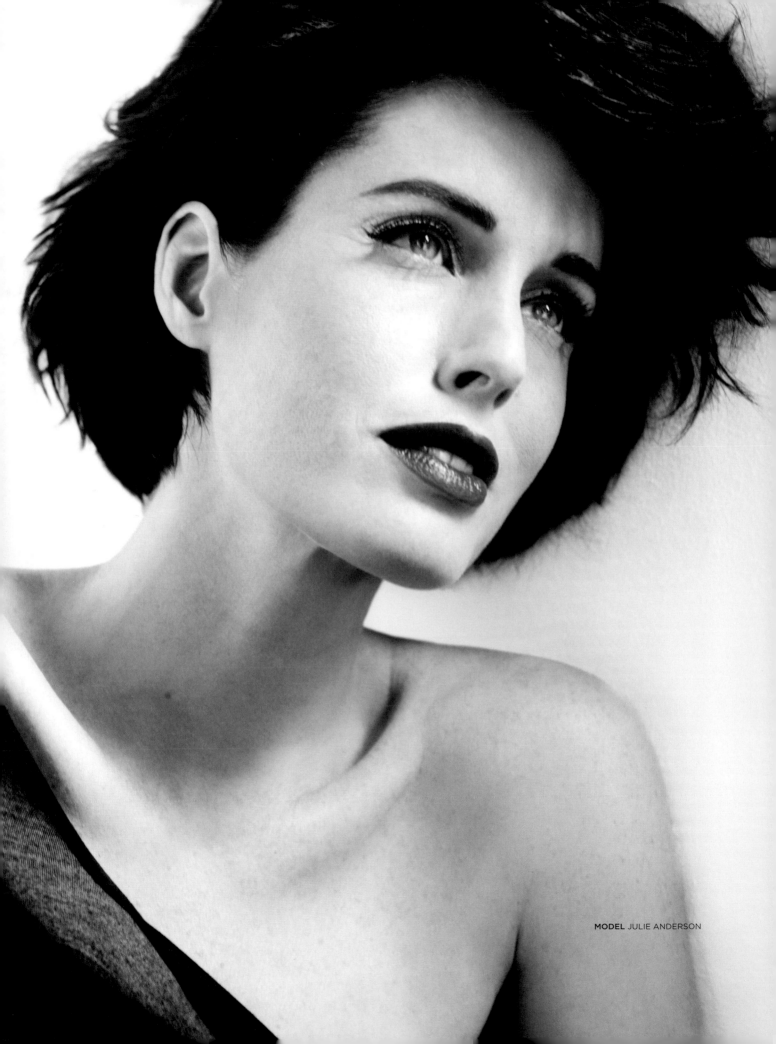

MODEL JULIE ANDERSON

Contents

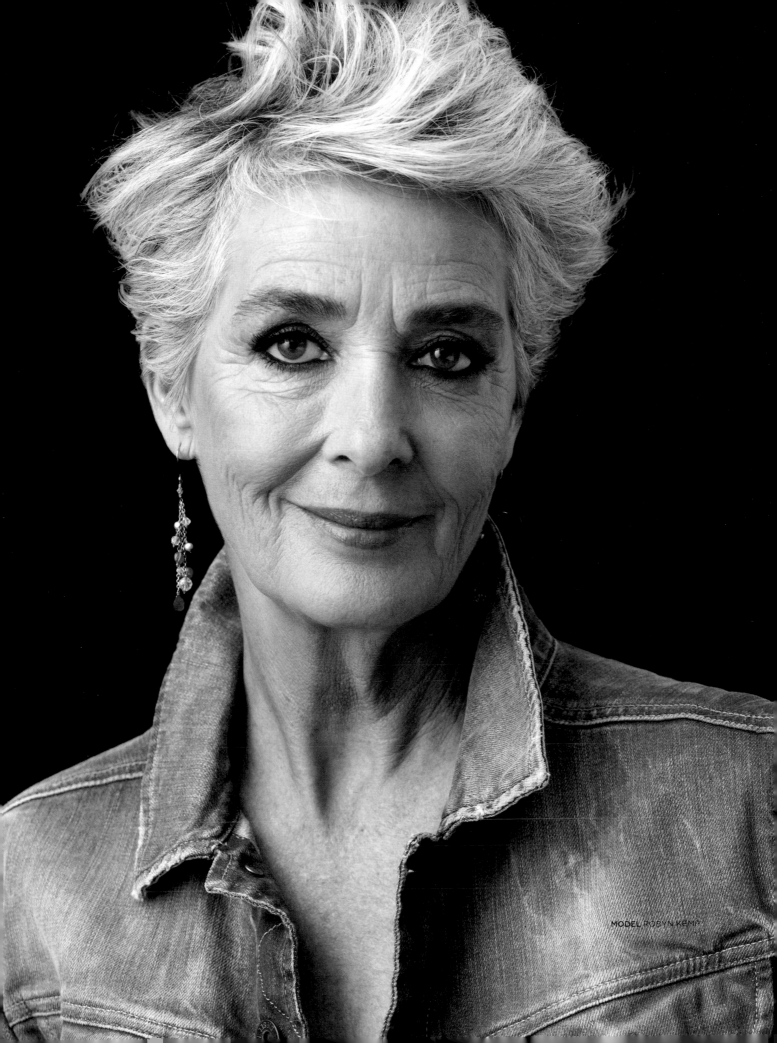

MODEL ROBYN KEMP

Introduction

I work with makeup every day, so I see how it can transform a woman's face. It's really frustrating to see women who could look so much more beautiful if they just got their makeup right. But it's not their fault—we can all pretty much blame our Mums, every girl's first makeup artist. By the time we're into our forties, we have a quarter-century habit learnt from our mothers. And we all know the hardest habit to break is a bad one.

That's why I'm so excited about this book, which will help make a difference to not only how you look, but also how you feel. It's not just about trying to hide lines and look like you did when you were 18—don't try to erase your life. What worked for you at 18 will simply not work for you at 40, and you'll just look silly if you try.

I've just turned 40, and it's really changed my perspective on how I want to look, and also what my look says about who I am. And that's what this book is about—classic, ageless beauty... something to embrace.

I'll apologise in advance—this book is about the brutal truth. You're going to face the facts about how you age, and how the right makeup can make all the difference in maintaining a timeless look that's more stunning than you ever imagined.

I'll start with the basics, which is all about getting your makeup kit right, as you can't create a masterpiece without the right tools. Then I'll talk colour—choosing the correct shade of foundation, using the right colours in the right place, contouring to accentuate or disguise your facial structure, and lots of secret tips that will revolutionise the way you do your makeup.

I have also created a series of classic 'day' and 'night' looks that will take ten years off in ten minutes, including easy to follow step-by-step instructions you can incorporate into your daily routine. These are the techniques and looks I use every day on some of the world's best models as well as myself and my friends.

I will also touch on the latest non-surgical cosmetic techniques that can correct a few flaws and enhance your look by improving your 'canvas'—your face.

This book is about the real world, about the challenges you encounter every day as you age, and what you can do to highlight your radiance and beauty regardless of your age. Through this book I hope to bring you completely into my world and share with you the secrets that will change not just the way you look, but also the way you feel every day. Welcome, and enjoy!

www.raemorris.com

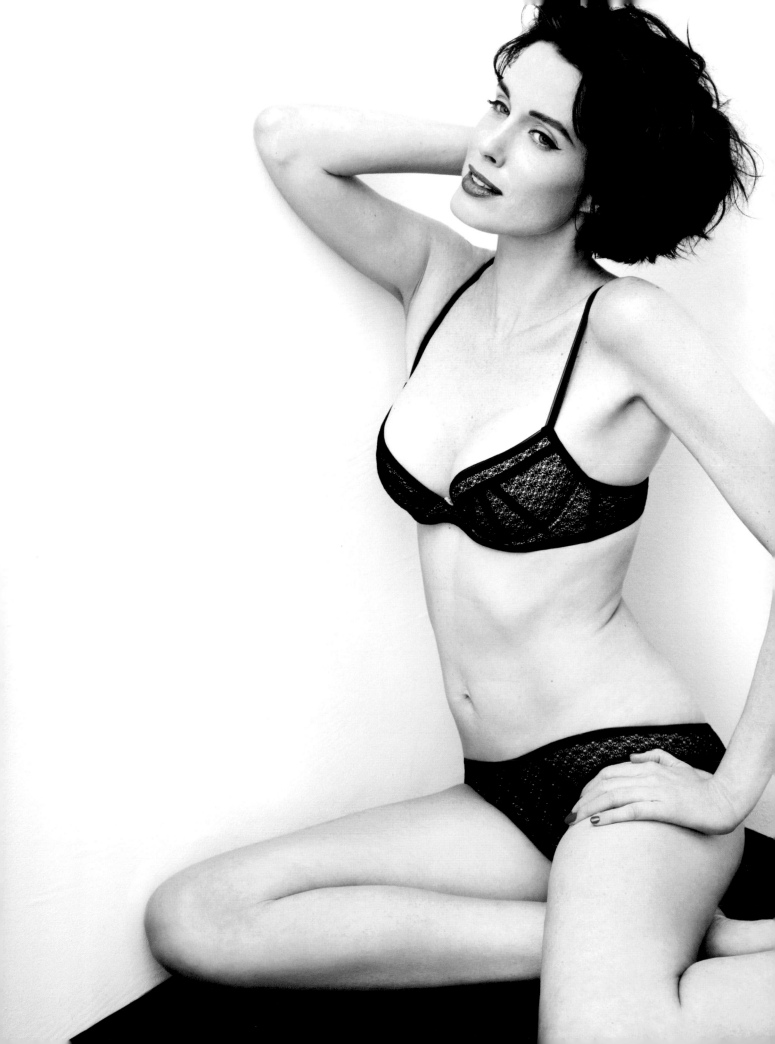

How you age

*F*irst, ageing is not a bad thing. It's kind of fabulous—a lot of people become much better looking as they get older. You don't want to peak too early! But there's a big difference between ageing and deteriorating (sorry, but I did warn you I would be blunt). Ageing is part of life, but how you do it, and how you feel and look, is up to you.

As you age, you'll experience some changes that are common to everyone, although some factors will depend on your genetic inheritance and lifestyle as well as the environment.

Here are some of the general signs of ageing.

- Temples become more concave.

- Hollows develop beneath the eyes and cheekbones.

- The jaw line becomes jowly and droopy.

- The neck becomes heavily lined, while the décolletage cops a continual beating from the elements. Depending on your age and skin type, your chest can become very red, freckled, lined and pigmented.

- Eyebrows become sparser and coarser, and lashes thinner.

- Earlobes droop.

- Hands become wrinkly, and veins and any signs of sun damage become more visible.

- Age spots appear on the hands and arms, which are often unflatteringly referred to as 'salami arms'—bet you won't be ordering that at the deli again!

Now before you get too depressed, save it— there's more to come...

- Pigmentation and age spots may appear on the face.

- The face may be constantly red as a result of broken capillaries and sun damage.

- The corners of the mouth droop.

- Eyelids become droopy.

- The brow bone becomes more pronounced, and the lips and the skin around the mouth lined.

Phew...how do you feel now? How effectively is the old 'I'm beautiful on the inside' line holding you together?

Now you may be genetically blessed and have none of these problems, but most of us have to take corrective measures to minimise the signs of ageing. Don't worry, it just comes down to:

- prevention;

- management, which includes treatment (see page 171) and illusion (refer to 'Beyond makeup', page 74); and, of course,

- makeup.

You should also be aware that there are some specific differences in the way men and women age—it's not a level playing field. For example, women age more than men in the chest area. This is because men have hair on their necks and chests, and every hair follicle contains an oil gland that keeps the skin soft and supple. Also, hair is a great sunscreen, which brings me to my next point—even when women apply sunscreen to their décolletage, what do they do next? That's right, they spray on perfume (pretty much pure alcohol), which immediately makes the sunscreen ineffective and dries out and thins their skin at the same time!

Look 10 years younger

There is so much you can do to make yourself look younger if you just get a few simple things right. But first you have to break the old habits that don't work for you any more and replace them with new ones that will instantly take years off how you look.

When I started thinking about this book, I paid even more attention to how older women do their makeup, dress and accessorise, and I couldn't help noticing that my attention was drawn to four key areas—the earlobes, décolletage, hands and mouth. These areas age obviously, and here is the epiphany I had... where do most women wear bling? Yes, on their earlobes, décolletage and hands. And if they throw on some bright red lipstick, they hit the jackpot, drawing attention to all the bits that give away their age the most.

Here's how you can use makeup to optimise the way you look—not only to disguise the signs of ageing but also to enhance your best features.

EYES

If you ever wear frosty white eye shadow, it just has to go. The '80s are over, and they just ain't coming back. This product is like putting a magnifying glass on problem areas and high-lighting them. Special effects makeup artists use it to make skin look more wrinkled, puffy and scaley. So just imagine what effect it will have on your appearance if you have puffy, heavy, hooded eyelids!

If you're lined around the eyes, use only rich, beautiful matte shades—definitely no shimmer!

Matching your eye shadow shade to your eye colour is so important—that's why we've put so much detail into the eye colour charts (see the section starting on page 44). Use these as your 'bible' when buying eye makeup.

You also have to let go of the fluorescent blues and glitter eyeliners if you use them. Think sophistication and elegance instead. And avoid old-school cream eye shadows altogether—they crease within seconds and give you oily eyelids.

As you age, your eyes become more watery, so you'll need to start using waterproof products, such as waterproof mascara, so your eye makeup doesn't run.

Eyelashes rock! As you get older, they tend to become sparser, but you can't let this happen. Now that you can get eyelash extensions that last up to six weeks, you don't need to apply mascara or attempt false lashes (see page 64).

Eyes tend to droop, which means the inner rim of the eye becomes more exposed. Therefore it's essential not to apply harsh eyeliner under your lower lash line, as this will accentuate any drooping and drag your eyes down even more.

As you age, your brow bone becomes more prominent and your lids become heavier and hooded, so arching your brows actually makes you look older (see page 54).

SKIN

As you get older, it's really important to avoid heavy, cakey foundation. And go easy on the powder, as it can make your skin look quite flat and dead. Your skin can lose its glow as you age, and you don't want to accentuate this, so stick with sheer translucent powders and steer clear of anything with beige or pink undertones, as these will age you ridiculously!

If your face is naturally a bit red, first apply a good foundation to disguise the redness and give you an even canvas to work on. Then apply the cheek colour in the right place, nice and high, to achieve that healthy, youthful look. Never smile when applying blush, because when you do so:

• your cheeks lift, so when you stop smiling your blush will be closer to your jaw; and

• your face wrinkles. If you apply blush to a wrinkled area, you won't get into the wrinkle creases, thus accentuating them. Applying blush while smiling is another technique makeup artists use to create lines, so make sure you avoid it.

Your makeup shouldn't stop with your face. For example, if you're wearing a low-cut dress, use a powdered mineral foundation on your décolletage, preferably one containing sunscreen—it will even out the skin beautifully and is perfect for the sensitive, finer skin in this region. And it's also less likely to rub off onto your clothes.

LIPS

Please make sure there are no eyebrows on your lips, ladies! Eyebrows should only be above your eyes. If there is even the hint of a stray hair anywhere else, get rid of it! Your tweezers should be your best friend.

If you have the luxury of beautifully shaped lips with minimal lines, you can choose any colour lipstick that suits your skin tone, but avoid anything glittery, frosty or metallic, as these actually accentuate wrinkling—your lips aren't a neon billboard! If you use a lip liner,

colour in the whole lip, don't just trace the outline. If you outline your lips, and colour in with a lipstick, the lipstick will wear off first, leaving the outline, and no one wants to look like Bobo the clown, do they?

Always test lipstick on your fingertip, which has the same texture and colour as your lip. Your fingertip has a blue-red tone, whereas the back of your hand (where most women test colours) is a neutral tone, so it will make the shade appear brighter and richer than when it is applied to your lips.

Use the 'one wipe test'—that is, one wipe of the lipstick to get the colour intensity you're after. If you have to do more than this, it's not the right lipstick for you. The more lipstick you put on, the more likely it is to run—remember, 'more on the mouth goes south'. (See also page 70.)

MEDICAL SOLUTIONS

With today's ever-changing technology, there is also a range of non-invasive medical procedures (see page 171) that can reduce the signs of ageing and significantly improve your 'canvas'.

At the end of the day, it's about feeling as good about yourself as you possibly can. Being confident in your appearance affects how you feel about yourself and therefore the way you face the world. It's that important.

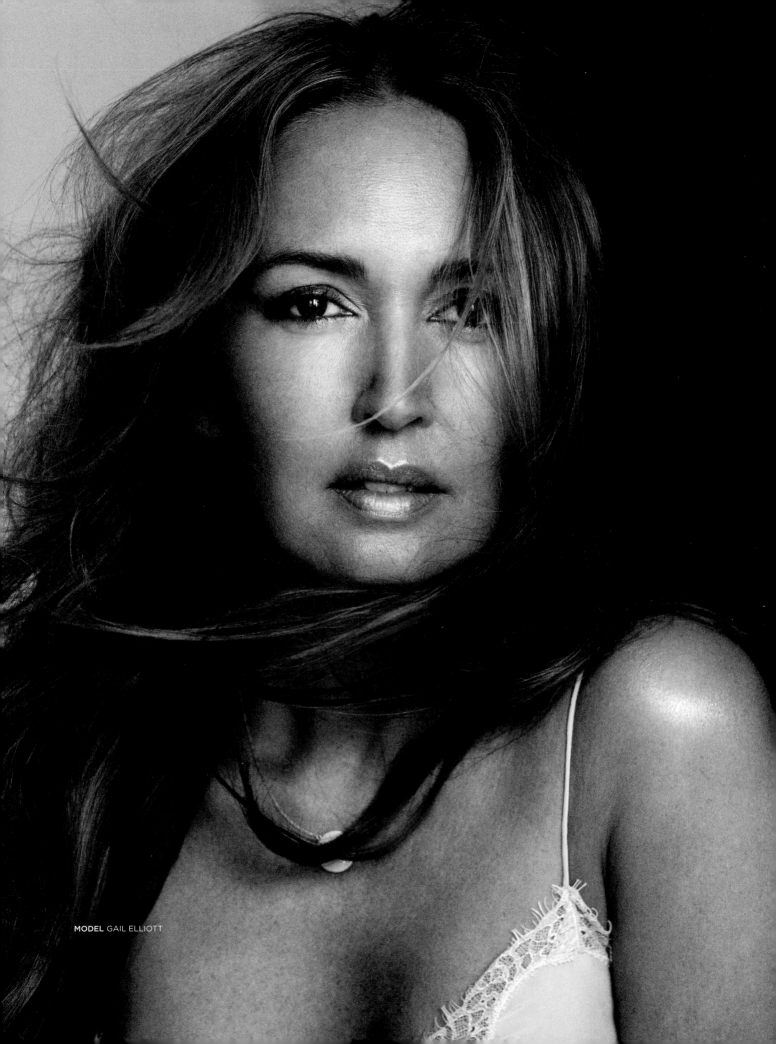
MODEL GAIL ELLIOTT

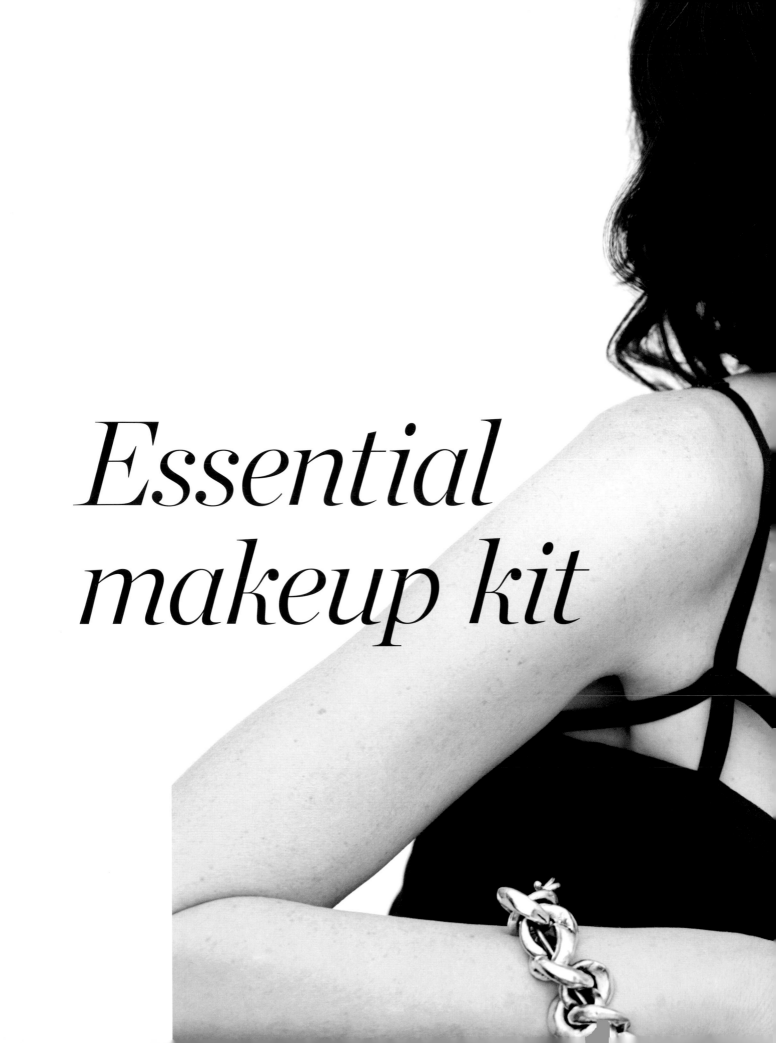

*Essential
makeup kit*

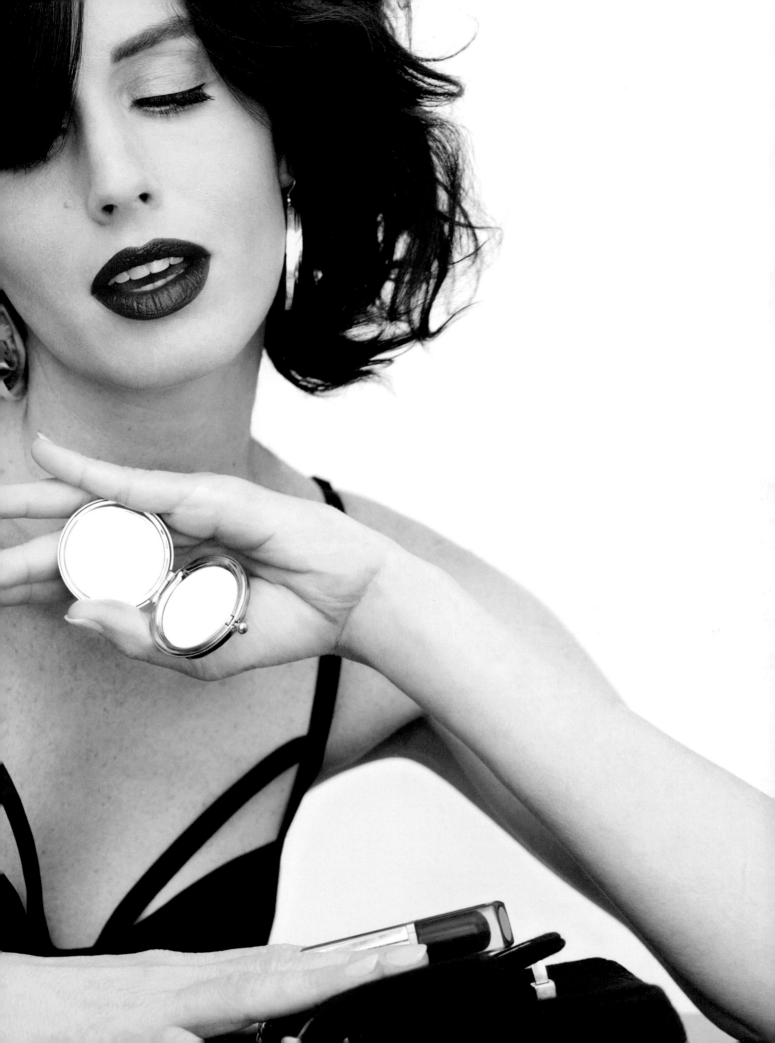

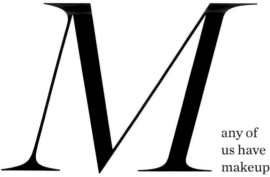

Many of us have makeup kits that are an assortment of bits and pieces and the odd application tool. Chances are most of the makeup will be either out of fashion or past its use-by date. If any of your makeup is more than two years old, throw it out!

The first step towards getting your makeup right is to have the right tools. It's better to buy a small range of the right makeup and spend less on disposable items such as lipstick, and use the money you've saved to invest in better brushes.

Good quality tools give you the control you need to do your makeup properly, and they'll last for years. I've spent decades searching the world for the best tools for my profession, but as I haven't always been able to find them, I've developed my own brush range. A brush must have the right fibres in the right density and shape. We'll cover this in detail in the brush section (see page 12), but to make it easier, visit www.raemorris.com to see what I use every day.

Keep it simple

As most women get older, they use fewer or no products on their face, or heaps more stuff than they've ever used before. To get the right look, and for a longer lasting makeup, you should simplify the products you use. Choosing one product that does it all—for example, a combined foundation, moisturiser and sunscreen—rather than several individual ones, makes it much easier (and quicker) to attain the final finish.

It's also worth looking for concentrated products—such as lipstick that goes on in one swipe, and rich black mascara that goes on with one stroke—so you can avoid multiple applications that create a 'caked on' effect.

Essential touch-up kit

Keep these key items in your handbag at all times so you can touch up your makeup when you're out and about.

- **Concealer** This comes in a small tube, so it's easy to carry. Think of it as concentrated foundation, the ultimate weapon for hiding the things you don't want others to see. Use a little on a small brush to hide blemishes and dark circles under your eyes, and to clean up any runny mascara or lipstick bleeds.

- **Foundation** If you have enough room in your bag, carry some foundation, otherwise just go with concealer. I put mine in a small container.

- **Blotting papers** These little miracles are great to have if you start to develop a 'greasy glow', as they'll remove all the shine, leaving your foundation untouched, and allowing you to refresh your makeup.

- **Eye pencil** Carry any eye pencil you may have used on the inner rim of your eyes (as the eyes water, they will need constant touching up).

- **Lipstick** Lipstick always fades, so it will need the occasional touch up.

- **Blush** It's better to put on the right amount of blush in the first place, then touch up all day, than to put on too much and hope it lasts the distance.

- **Hand cream** Keep your hands soft and supple with regular applications of hand cream.

- **Sunscreen** Always use sunscreen on your face, hands and chest. Imagine attending an outdoor wedding reception without any sun protection—a beetroot-red face is not a good look, especially when you're wearing a glamorous red frock!

Full makeup kit

Now let's talk about the makeup kit essentials that you keep at home. On the following pages you'll find all you need, from blotting papers and primers to lipsticks and eyelash curlers.

FACE AND BODY SCRUB

Seriously, the best facial/body scrub in the world is so exclusive, you can't buy it retail! It also happens to be the cheapest—you just make it yourself. Simply mix together equal parts of bicarbonate of soda and any good quality water-based cleanser you can buy from your pharmacy.

For your face, use about half a teaspoon of each; for your whole body, increase it to a handful of each. Combine it with a bit of warm water and you're ready to go. This is the mix recommended by many dermatologists as a gentle, non-reactant exfoliant, so don't be afraid to get between your eyebrows and over your lips.

Exfoliate your skin no more than once a week, and do not exfoliate at all if you are using chemical peeling creams or any products that contain AHAs, Retin As or BHAs, as these remove the upper layers of your skin. Using an exfoliant would be overkill, plus it would damn well hurt! If you're receiving treatment from a dermatologist, always check with him or her before using any exfoliant.

BABY WIPES

Use non-alcoholic, non-perfumed baby wipes, which contain few or no chemicals, so there's less risk of skin reactions. I use them daily to help remove oil before I start applying makeup, and also to help clean up any flakes of eye shadow that drop under the eyes.

BLOTTING PAPERS

These are great if you have oily skin or tend to perspire excessively. Make sure you buy the non-powdered version, otherwise they'll change the colour of your foundation. If you like to powder your foundation, blot your skin first to remove excess oil before powdering, as it's the build-up of oil that creates the 'cakey' look. It's simple—the less oil on your skin, the less powder will stick.

MAKEUP PRIMER

This is basically a moisturiser that contains extra silicone and glycerine, which levels out any uneven skin texture, allowing you to apply foundation a lot more evenly. If you're going to use a primer, don't use a moisturiser, because you'll just be doubling up. Using more than one product under foundation won't allow your skin to absorb it, so it will separate and look patchy.

I recommend water-based primers because, as you'll see, all the foundations I prefer are water-based and mix together beautifully. You can also get 'anti-red' primers that help reduce redness.

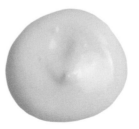

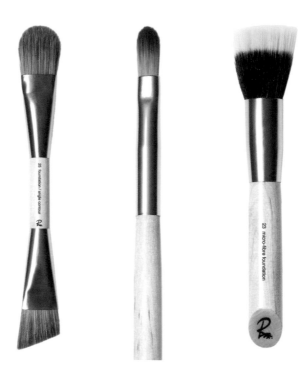

BRUSHES

You don't have to spend lots of money on makeup brushes. For top quality brushes in my ultimate brush roll, go to my website (www.raemorris.com) and buy them online. To test a brush you already have, stand it on its tip on the back of your hand—if the bristles collapse, replace the brush.

Double-ended foundation brush

The rounded end of the Foundation/Angle Contour brush is great for applying liquid-based foundation, while the angled end is perfect for contouring with cream- or grease-based products. The bristles don't absorb much product, thus reducing wastage.

Concealer brush

Use the Concealer Brush to apply all types of concealers, especially to the under-eye area. Its non-absorbent bristles minimise product wastage. You can also use it as a lip brush and to apply liquid or grease-based eye shadows for the wet lid look.

Foundation brush

The fantastic Micro-fibre Foundation brush makes liquid and mineral/powder foundation look flawless. The white fibres absorb the foundation while the black ones polish it in, so you don't need to keep loading up with product. To create the illusion of a thinner leg, use it with body highlighter but only apply a stroke down the front of the leg. You can also use it to even out a fake tan or to apply a wash of foundation to your hands and feet in order to reduce the visibility of veins.

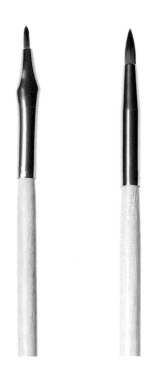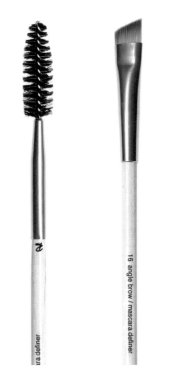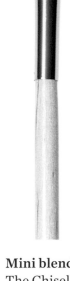

Eyeliner brushes
Designed for the finest eye-liners, the hook on the Precision Bent-liner (above left) makes it easy to apply liquid or gel eyeliner to the inner corner of the eye while you steady your hand on the face. It can also be used for very fine concealing, or to create the finest brow hairs and under-eye lashes. Use the Perfect Eyeliner brush (above right) to apply fine- to medium-width eyeliner (think Audrey Hepburn) or to create beauty spots. It's also a great brush to use for precision concealing.

Combined mascara wand/angle brush
This is my number one brush, and I couldn't do makeup without it. Use the Mascara Definer to apply mascara and groom your eyebrows. Use the Angle end to apply the perfect eyeliner flick, to apply fine hair strokes to the sparse areas of the brow, and to define your brow (it's perfect for tapering off the brow line). If your lipstick starts to bleed, dip the angled end in some foundation, then retrace the outline of your lips.

Mini blending brush
The Chiselled Smudger is perfect for blending or smudging eye shades or gels close to the lash line. It's also great for softening or smudging liquid eyeliner or for any other intricate work around the eyes—its compact size helps keep your eye shadow perfectly in place.

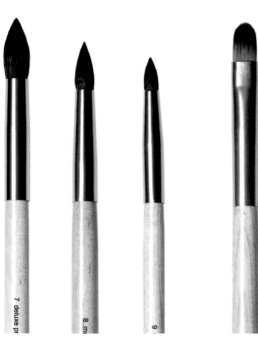

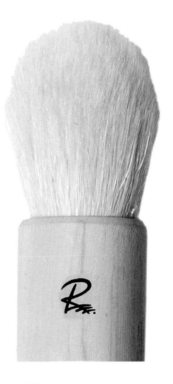

Eye shadow blending brushes
Having only one blending brush just won't cut it. I've personally designed three sizes—the Deluxe Precision, Medium Precision and Detail Precision Shaders. The Deluxe is the one you'll use the most—from full eye shading to precision shading—while the Medium is a great all-round blending eye brush, and the Detail is perfect for blending a smoky eye, especially around sensitive eyes.

Lip brush
If you use my firm synthetic Lip Brush, which is slightly longer and stronger than the standard lip brush, you'll avoid those unwanted stray brush hairs that ruin your lip line. Also, a synthetic brush doesn't absorb as much product, so more lipstick ends up on your lips. This brush does double duty as a concealer brush.

Kabuki brush
I could not do my job without the Deluxe Kabuki, a little miracle brush. You'll see this brush used extensively throughout this book. It's like a ball of cotton wool and does just about everything, from powdering to applying cream blush, bronzer and highlighter. You can also use it to contour and blend eye shadow, as well as enhance and define a cleavage line, all without leaving awful brush marks. You should have at least two.

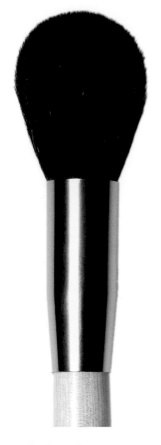

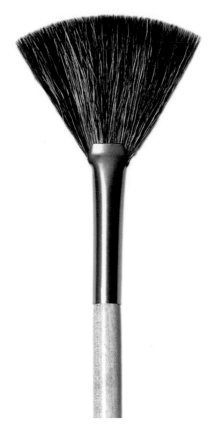

Powder brush

I mainly use the Pro Powder brush if I'm powdering the whole face, applying shimmer to the body or, rarely, as a substitute for a kabuki brush. Use it to apply both powder and bronzer to the face and body.

Fan brush

Great for removing messy eyelash fallout, the Fan Highlighter is designed to apply highlighter to the cheekbone, the centre of the forehead and the collar bone. I sometimes use it to fill in fine hair lines or temple areas. Just use it with an eye shadow that matches your hair colour.

A great idea is to buy a stack of small clear jars, then fill them with all your little essentials (for example, concealer and blush). That way you'll have everything you need on standby, and they take up hardly any space!

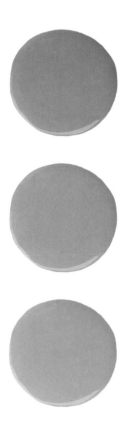

FOUNDATION

This is the most essential product in your makeup kit, but the one many women overlook. Of all the makeup products, foundation is the one that can make you look the most youthful. There is a full chapter on prepping and foundation coming up (see page 22), but in terms of your kit, you may need two to three shades of foundation so you can match its colour to your skin tone all year round—summer, winter and whenever you use fake tan.

The various types of foundation offer several types of coverage, so for:

- **stunning skin** with no blemishes, go for sheer, light textures, preferably water-based;
- **skin with subtle blemishes** or some slight pigmentation, choose sheer to medium coverage; and
- **problem skin**, choose medium to high coverage. Remember, if you use the right brush to apply a heavier foundation, it will look air-brushed and be hard to detect.

CONCEALER

Your makeup kit just isn't complete without a concealer, because as you age there are more things you need to cover up. Opt for liquid or cream concealers, as they are flexible and move with your skin. Stay away from products with heavy, cakey, powdery textures.

FACE POWDERS

These come in two basic forms—compressed and translucent. Look for the lightest powders in the same shade or one to two shades lighter than your base. They should have the sheerest texture so they don't change the colour of your foundation. Face powders should be invisible on your skin. Keep away from shimmery forms, as they will only enhance lines.

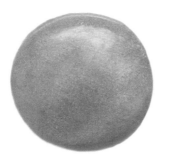

BLUSH

There are two types of blush—cream and powder—and each comes in either a matte or a shimmery finish (so there are four options in total). I love cream blush because it's easier to blend. Rubbing a cream blush into your skin with a kabuki brush gets right into all the lines.

Use powder blush only on top of powder foundation and/or face powder, and cream blush only on top of liquid or cream foundation. You'll notice that I do use powdered blush quite a bit in the Looks section (see pages 82–169), which is fine if the cheeks are relatively free of lines and powdered first, in which case either type is appropriate. If you're lined, stick to cream blush.

CONTOURING CREAM OR SHADOW

Use this product to create cheekbones and give your cheeks, eyes and jaw line more definition (see page 34). Contouring products aren't for everyone, but they can make a massive difference if they're used correctly. There are two types—powder and cream or grease. I only use the matte shadows (the same ones I use on eyebrows) or dark foundations in a grease form (which should be at least three to four shades darker than your natural skin).

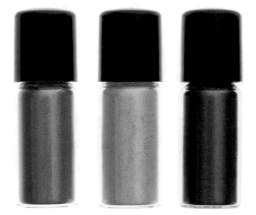

HIGHLIGHTERS

Use these to highlight your skin and eyes. The two essential eye colours are gold and silver, and you should make your choice based on the jewellery you wear—if you prefer silver jewellery, for example, choose silver highlighter. Other areas I highlight include the top of the lip and, if you have great skin texture, the cheekbones.

If you have beautiful skin, you can also add luminisers, the liquid versions of highlighters, to your liquid foundation for an all-over glow. I've applied this technique to Leona Edmiston's face (see page 30) so you can see the effect.

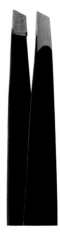 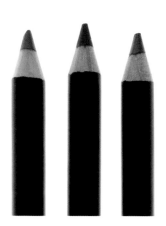 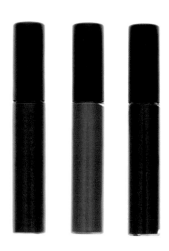

TWEEZERS

I prefer pointed tweezers because you can remove every hair in sight with them and also define the brow beautifully. Remember, you're only meant to have brows above your eyes—any hair above your lip has to go! Always use your tweezers on an angle so you don't stab yourself, especially if you're using sharp pointed tweezers. And make sure your tweezers grip hairs properly. When you need to resharpen them, use a metal nail file.

To clean tweezers, simply wipe them with a cotton bud dipped in antiseptic or brush cleaner.

BROW PENCIL

Next to foundation, your eyebrows are the most important part of your makeup regimen, and getting them right can change your entire look (see page 54). Choose a brow pencil that matches your brow hair colour (sounds obvious, I know, but it's a common mistake).

BROW MASCARA

I have used the amazing little secret of brow mascara throughout this book to temporarily conceal grey regrowth in eyebrows and on hairlines. It's rare and hard to find, but great for temporarily lightening or darkening your brows, covering grey and matching the colour of your brows to your hair colour.

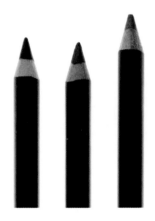

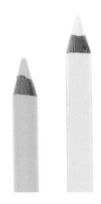

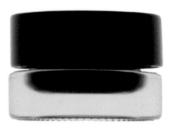

KOHL PENCILS

There are two types of kohl pencil—waterproof and non-waterproof. For the inner rim, use a non-waterproof pencil, as this area of the eye is wet and waterproof pencils won't work. As you get older, your eyes tend to water more, and there are also more creases in the eye area, so make sure any pencil you use around your eye is a non-waterproof one. Avoid shimmery ones.

WHITE OR CREAM PENCILS

These are great for disguising redness in the inner rim of the eye, opening the eye and making you look instantly younger! If they're waterproof, they won't work on the wet inner rim.

BLACK PENCIL

This should not be waterproof, so you can apply it to the inside of the eye for those glamorous occasions. It also works well as a smudged eyeliner on the top lash line. In cold weather you can heat up the pencil by rubbing it on the back of your hand. This will release the pigment and soften the pencil, giving it a crayon-like feel and improving the intensity of the colour.

EYELINER

There are two types of eyeliner—liquid and gel. Liquid eyeliner is great if you're skilled at applying it. But on older eyelids the skin moves a lot, and liquid eyeliner tends to crack, so it will be harder to use. For this reason, and because you only get one chance to nail an eyeliner, I always recommend the gel type. It's easy to use, and doesn't dry as quickly as liquid eyeliner, so you have more time to blend. And once a gel eyeliner dries, it's waterproof.

Always apply gel eyeliner quickly with a sharp-angled or liner brush.

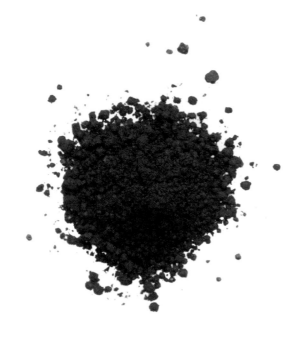

EYE SHADOWS

Two to three shades of eye shadow sounds pretty basic, but you'll be amazed how much you can achieve with so little. Stay away from the frosty and shimmery eye shadows, as these will enhance any lines you may have.

When you're buying eye shadow, use a clean fingertip and wipe over the product once, then look at the intensity (I call this the 'one wipe trick'). If the colour isn't as intense on your finger as it looks in the package, don't buy it. It's better to have a strong, intense colour that you can soften with loose translucent powder or good blending.

Never use generic cream eye shadows, as there is so much oil on the eyelids to begin with, and cream eye shadows will crease in seconds! But new-technology cream shadows on the market dry like eye shadow and last for eight hours—these are the only ones to use.

EYELASH CURLERS

As you get older, you'll have a lot fewer eyelashes, so it's even more important to make the most of them! Don't spend hours doing a fabulous eye, then leave your lashes looking like straight fence posts. If your eyelashes don't have a natural curl, use a manual eyelash curler (pictured on the left) before you apply mascara.

If you haven't used an eyelash curler before, and the mere thought of it terrifies you, use a heated one either before or after mascara. The manual version can pinch your eyelids if it's not used correctly, so only use it if you're a pro, and *before* applying mascara.

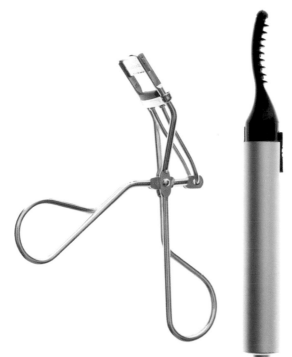

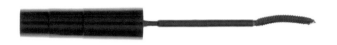

MASCARA

I mostly use only waterproof black mascara. Waterproof mascara does not break your eyelashes—that's just a myth—but you do have to be more careful when removing it, as it's a lot harder than any standard mascara. Just use a waterproof eye makeup remover (or oil if you're stuck). Always go for a metal 'comb' mascara applicator, such as the one I've personally designed—once you use one, you'll never want to use a wand again.

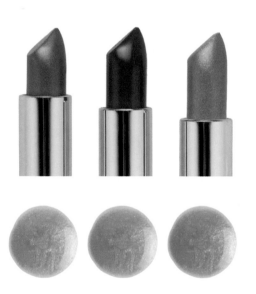

LIPSTICK AND LIP GLOSS

As you age, a lot more lines will develop around your mouth, so minimise the use of thick, gluey glosses on your lips. Choose lipstick shades you love after only one application. Lipstick is wax-based, so if you use too much on your lips, it will run once it heats up. Instead, go for less product and more colour intensity.

If your lips are excessively lined, avoid lipstick altogether. Use tinted lip balms in soft, nude rose shades instead, and concentrate on your eye makeup. Also, if you're going to draw attention to your lips, make sure you remove any hair that shouldn't be there.

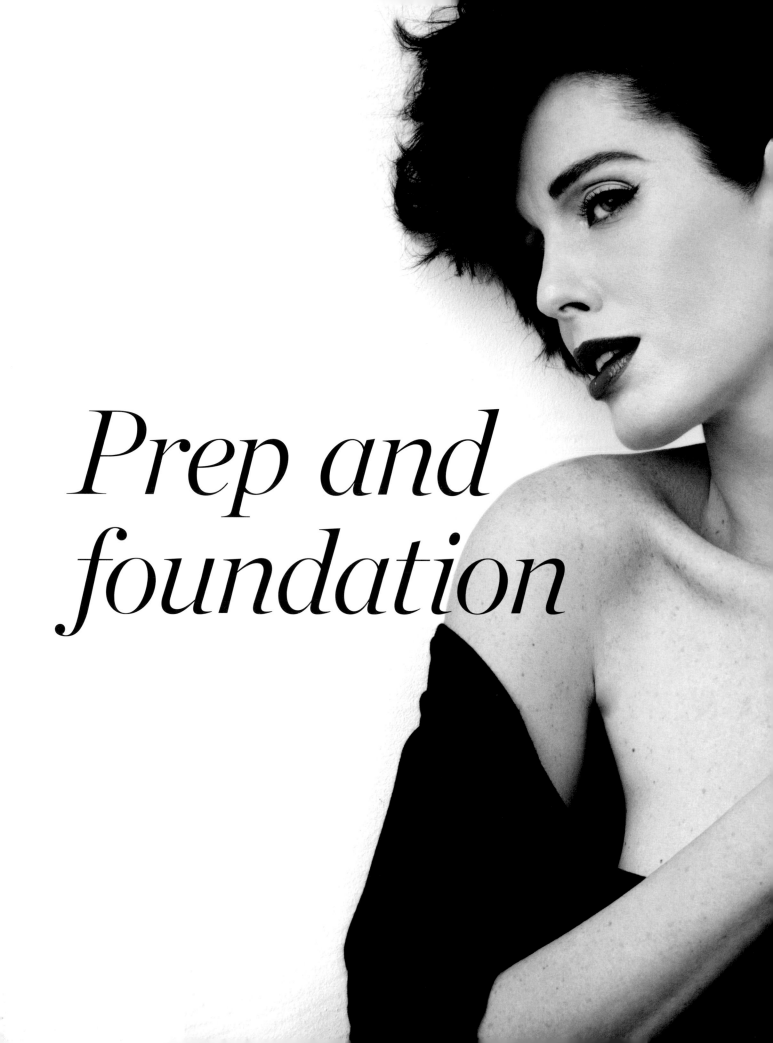

Prep and foundation

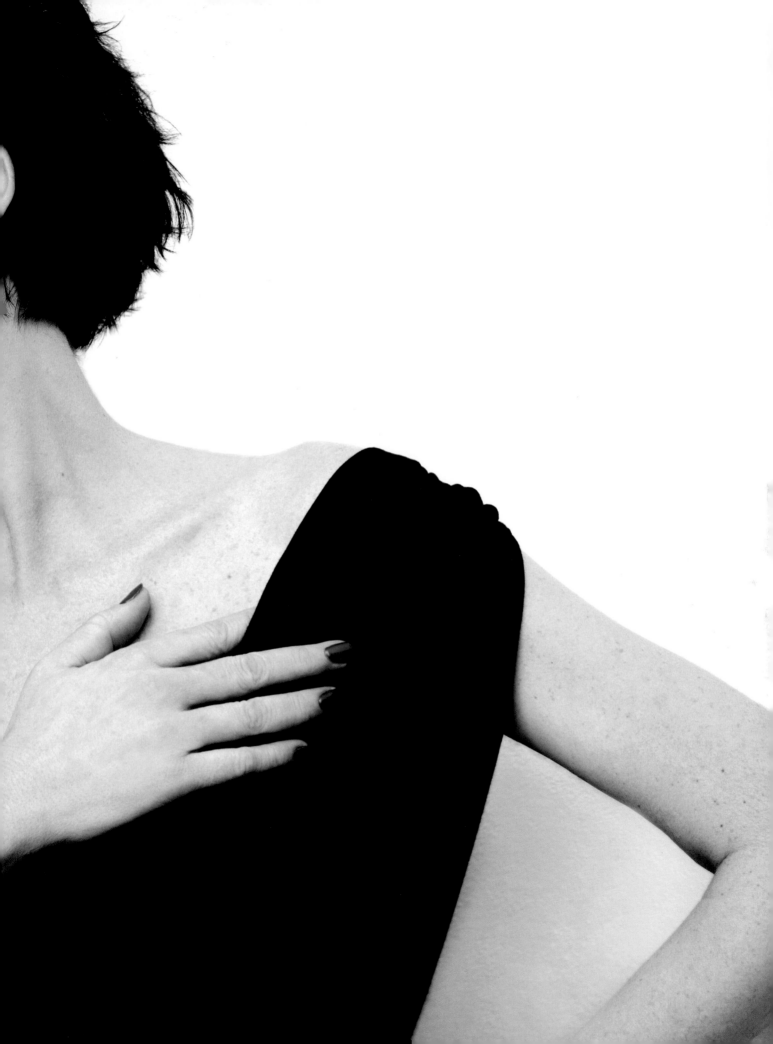

S kin preparation or prepping is the makeup stage that most women avoid so they can get to the fun colour stuff, but it's the crucial step in determining how long your makeup will last and how easy it will be to apply and maintain. This can make the difference between a great night out and one constantly interrupted by trips to the bathroom!

Prepping comprises three steps—cleansing, moisturising (or priming) and applying foundation (which includes concealing) and maybe powder. Get the first two steps right and you'll have the perfect foundation to create a long-lasting look that will be easy to maintain. As you age, your skin texture becomes more uneven, so prepping becomes even more important.

Older women tend to use too many face creams—for example, multiple moisturisers and eye creams—so they become over-moisturised! By this I mean that their skin becomes 'clogged', so their makeup cannot be absorbed, and what they put on top of their foundation will probably slide off. When you're applying makeup, the rule is to have only one product between you and your foundation (sometimes you don't even need that). The more cream on your face before you apply foundation, the harder it is for your makeup to stick.

When it comes to selecting prepping products, there are two rules.

1 Use either water- or oil-based products, never both. Oil and water don't mix, and combining incompatible products is the main reason makeup doesn't last.

2 Pick products you won't react to. I prefer products that are perfume-free, and my general rule is that if it's not recommended for use on sunburnt or extremely sensitive skin, don't use it—ever!

Cleansing

It's important not to use anything that leaves a film on your skin, so cleanse your skin with a pH-balanced product—for the pH to match your skin, it should have a reading of 4.5 to 5.5.

Non-alcoholic, non-perfumed baby wipes will change your life! Not only will they remove all the oil from your skin, but they will also leave no residue, so you can go straight to the next step—great if you're not in a position to wash your face with a cleanser as you normally would, or if you're nowhere near running water.

Priming or moisturising

You don't always have to use a toner—I never do. But if your skin is oily, use it only in the T-zone. If your skin is extra-oily, use moisturiser only in select areas, such as on the cheekbones and lips. Remember, the golden rule for using skin products is to use only one product underneath your foundation. Foundation needs to disappear 'into' the skin, not sit on top of it. (Imagine how much money I've just saved you!)

If you're in a mad rush, a toner can cleanse your skin very well. Just make sure it is a gentle, pH-based formula and doesn't leave a residue, as this will affect your makeup.

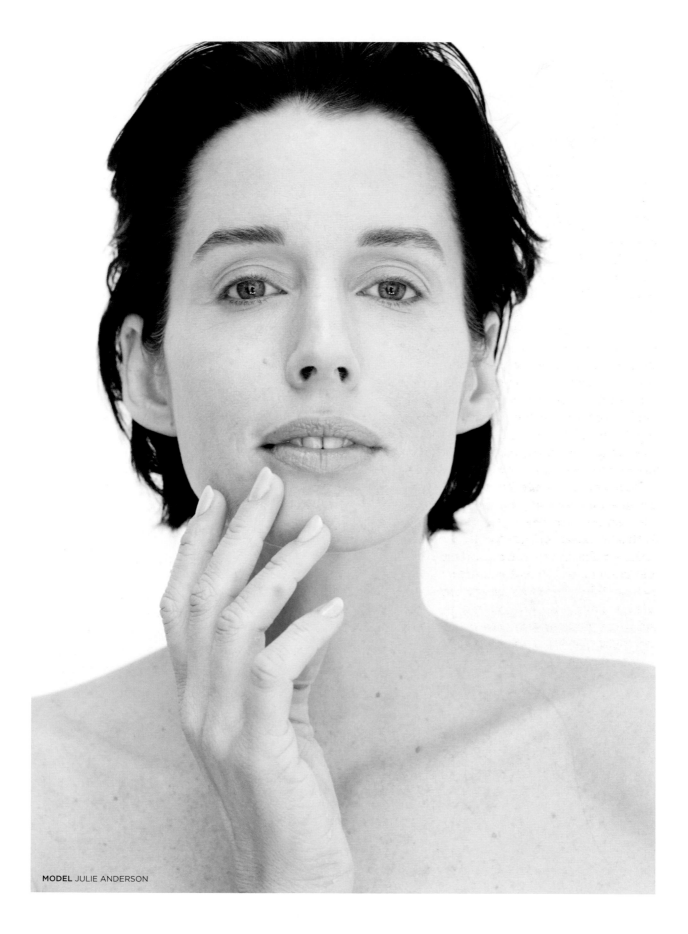

MODEL JULIE ANDERSON

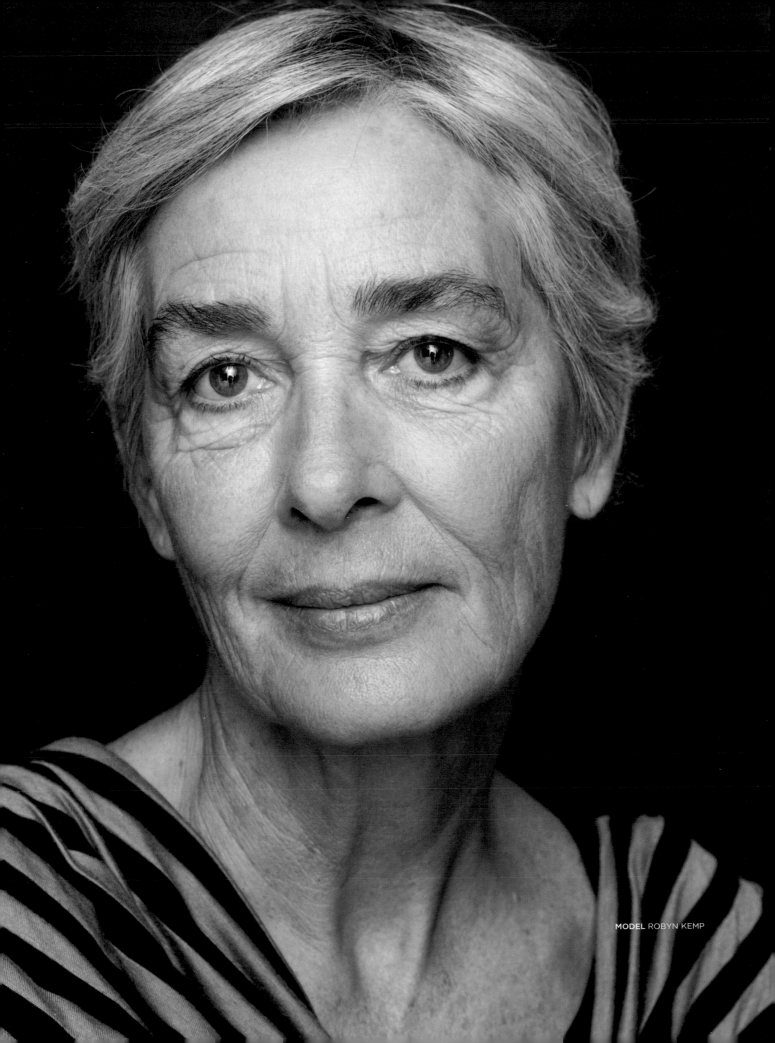

MODEL ROBYN KEMP

Don't moisturise your eyelids, because, as I keep saying, this is one of the greasiest parts of your face. Now wipe your finger over your eyelid—see what I mean? The biggest killer for eye makeup is oil, either your own or from a moisturiser. It's simply impossible to blend eye shadow on an oily eyelid.

If someone's skin is oily, I might not use a moisturiser at all. Remember that most foundations now contain moisturiser, so make sure you don't overdo it.

Anti-ageing skincare tips

While this isn't a skincare book, there are some really simple things you can do to reduce the signs of ageing.

1 EXFOLIATING

Exfoliating removes dead layers of skin and gives you a fresh base to work with, but you should only exfoliate every week or so. My favourite exfoliant is bicarbonate of soda mixed with cleansing lotion. For more on exfoliating, see page 11.

2 SUNSCREEN

If you spend a lot of time outside, apply a sunscreen under your foundation, or use a product that combines the two. Remember to choose the least greasy sunscreen so your makeup will have as much 'grip' as possible.

3 DÉCOLLETAGE AND NECK

There are two reasons why women age faster than men in this area. To find out why, go back to page 4.

4 HANDS AND FEET

If you have dry hands and/or feet, here's a fantastic tip. Before you go to bed, smother your hands and feet in pure lanolin, then put on cotton gloves (you can buy them from any pharmacy) and socks. In the morning your hands and feet will be back in the land of the living.

Now you're ready to apply some foundation and concealer!

Foundation

The key to a youthful look is skin that glows, something you lose as you age. You also develop blemishes such as age spots, and your skin tone becomes uneven (but at least it's better than the acne you may have had as a teenager!). Foundation and concealer are the keys to evening out everything and providing the perfect stage for your makeup to perform.

If you have an amazing base foundation, something as simple as mascara and blush is enough. I don't understand why some women don't wear foundation—the more uneven your skin, the more you need. Don't worry about how foundation feels, it's how it looks that's important (if it looks spectacular, you'll soon get used to how it feels). Your skin is porous, so that initial heavy feeling you may experience after applying foundation will fade and, besides, so what? High heels aren't comfortable, but you wouldn't go to a party in 'sensible' shoes, would you?

If you want to look like a celebrity on the red carpet or a model in a magazine, you have to use the products they use in the way they use them—it's that simple. The right foundation, even if it feels thick, will not *look* thick if it's applied correctly with the right brush. Your body heat will actually help your skin absorb it, and therefore thin it down.

TYPES OF FOUNDATION

Foundations come in a number of forms. Simply choose the one that suits you best.

1 Sheer tinted foundation This type provides you with minimal coverage but is great if you have dry skin. Buy one with an added sunscreen—extra bonus!

2 Mineral powder foundation This not only looks wonderful, but is also terrific for your skin. Most minerals contain sunscreen but give you a powdery matte finish, so only use them if that's the look you're trying to achieve.

3 Creamy liquid foundation Ranging from light to heavy coverage, this type is my favourite because it's very flexible and gives the skin a dewy glow. If you have lines, it won't 'crack', and it's really easy to reapply during the course of the day (which you can't really do with a powdered foundation).

Translucent powder

I never like using powder without foundation beneath because it doesn't provide any coverage, even though it's great for matteing down oily skin. So if you use translucent powder on its own, you'll still have the redness, pigment and uneven skin tone you started with. All you'll achieve is to make your uneven skin texture look dryer and matte, and this can actually make you look older.

However, translucent powder is fabulous on top of foundation, as it gives the skin a velvety finish. I use it extensively throughout this book. It is also the essential tool to use on your eyelids before you apply eye shadow, as it will not only make blending easier but also make your eye shadow look amazing.

Concealer

You must have this miracle product in your makeup kit! Your concealer, which comes in liquid and grease forms, should be one shade paler than your foundation and provide you with great coverage.

Now remember, the colours you're trying to conceal are the dark purple-blue shade you tend to get beneath and in the corner of your eyes; dark brown age spots and pigmentation; and forms of redness, such as broken capillaries, scars and sun damage.

The best way to test a concealer is to see if it covers dots made by red and blue ink pens on the back of your hand. It must erase them, with little or no trace of product—it's better to see the hint of a scar than to apply too much concealer. On the other hand, you should buy a strong concealer that will give you full coverage. You'll use less, and you can always thin it down with a hint of moisturiser if you need to.

You can also use concealer on the parts of your skin that are starting to 'sink'—for example, your temples and cheeks. Even if you don't need to conceal anything, it's a great way to lighten and lift areas that have started to recede.

Skin texture

Now I'm going to show you the different types of foundation and how they appear on the skin. Refer to the photographs of fashion designer Leona Edmiston on the next few pages.

SHEER TINTED FOUNDATION

We haven't photographed this type, as it just doesn't cut it for women over the age of 35. It allows too much of your natural skin to show through, so it's really part of the skincare family of products. Don't expect any coverage—it just lightly evens out your skin tone. Most sheer foundations combine a sunscreen, moisturiser and foundation. They are perfect for healthy skins and for women of a certain age who have flawless skin and don't like to wear foundation.

NATURAL FOUNDATION

This is my favourite, the one I prefer to use on everybody. With a natural creamy/liquid foundation, you can achieve a range of coverage, from sheer to high, depending on its strength. It is also the most versatile because you can choose the coverage level by diluting it with water-based moisturiser—it will give you a dewy finish, but you can also matte it down with powder. It will last longer too.

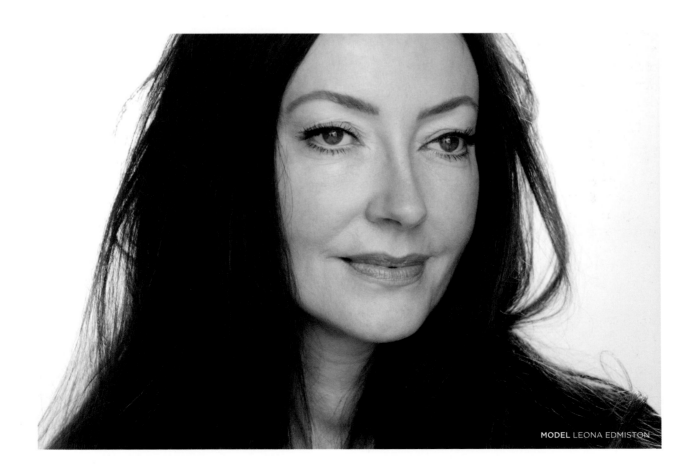

MODEL LEONA EDMISTON

DEWY FOUNDATION

To achieve a more luminous, dewy glow, add creamy gold or (if you're already tanned) bronze shimmery liquid to your current foundation. This is fabulous on youthful, blemish-free skin. I occasionally use this on women who are over 40 but only if they are blemish-free. You do have to be careful, as it can accentuate wrinkles. If that's your concern, highlight areas that tend to be free of wrinkles, regardless of your age.

In this shot I have highlighted the corners of Leona's eyes, the top of the lip, the upper cheekbones, the centre of the eyelids, and down the bridge of the nose.

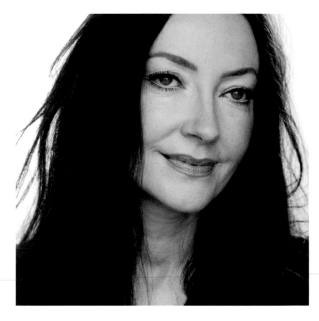

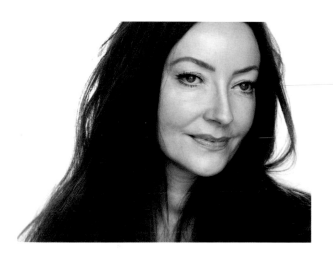

VELVETY FOUNDATION

Velvety is one down from matte, between a creamy texture and matte, and not quite as flat-looking. For this texture, apply liquid foundation and then translucent powder over the top—you shouldn't be able to detect the powder. Translucent powders are fabulous because they're so fine. All they really do is tone down excessive shine. If you're using powder during the day and you want to touch up your makeup, use blotting papers to blot off excess oil before you reapply.

Powder mineral foundations, if fine enough, will produce the same finish.

MATTE FOUNDATION

There are two ways to achieve this texture. One is to apply your liquid foundation as you normally would, then use a heavier matte type of powder all over. These powders are thicker, with no trace of shimmer, and matte down shine completely. Most women use matte powders to make their makeup last longer, which it may do, but it also makes them look four times older!

The other is to use a matte all-in-one version, like a mineral foundation, but I find this texture quite ageing on women whose skin is extremely dry or heavily lined.

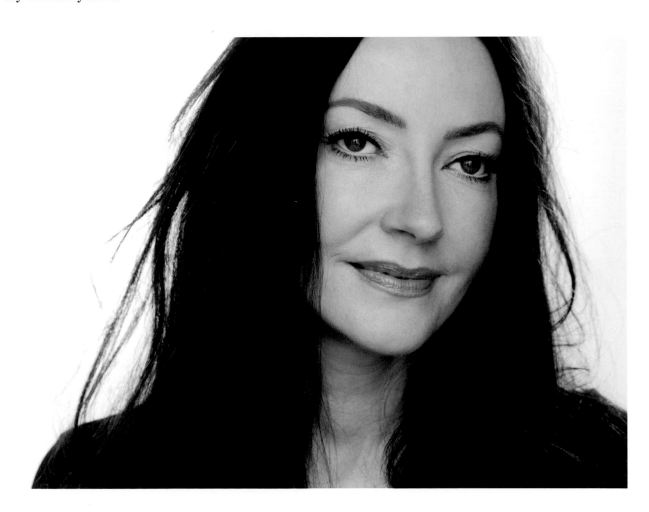

Contouring

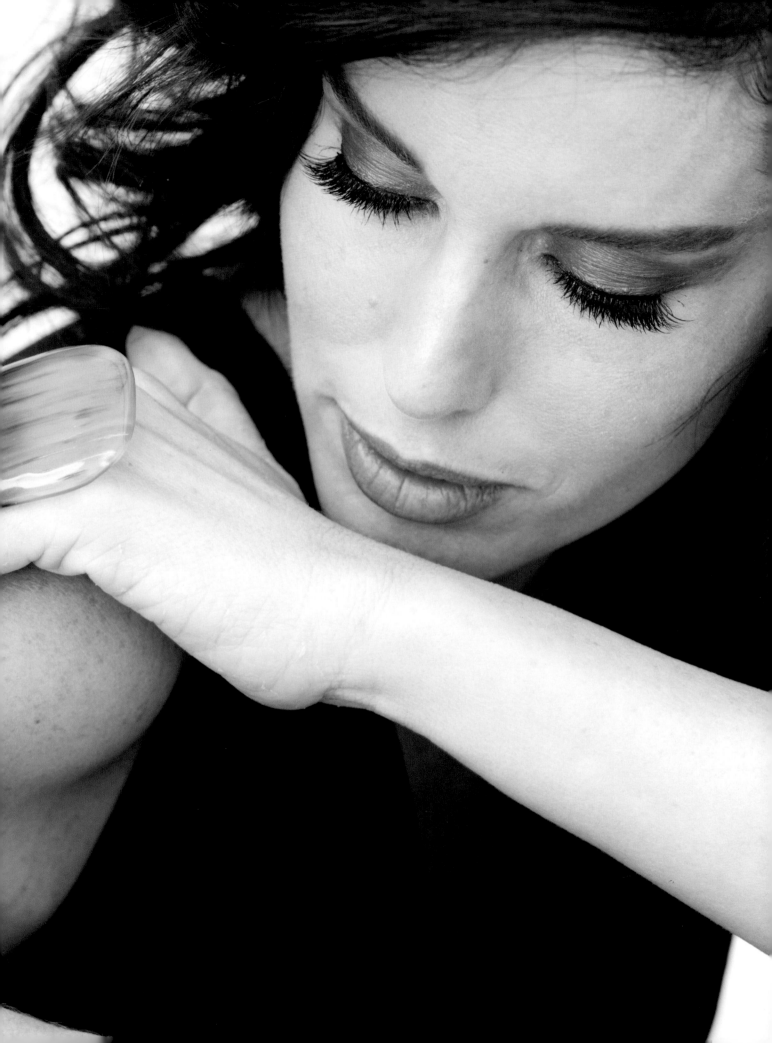

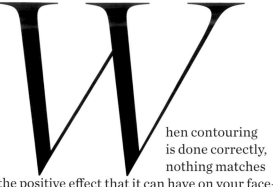

When contouring is done correctly, nothing matches the positive effect that it can have on your face—it can literally be as powerful as a facelift!

Contouring is where you use a product (either a foundation or an eye shadow) that's three to four shades darker than your natural skin tone to create the illusion of a shadow, thus increasing the definition of your facial features. Placing a 'shadow' in one area has the effect of highlighting (or raising) the areas on either side, such as cheek bones.

I'm going to show you which facial features you can use for contouring, but you need to be careful. Depending on your facial structure and features, not all of these areas may be suitable for you.

For contouring, all women fall into one of these three categories:

1 those who need to define their features more—for example, creating the illusion of stronger cheekbones for those with a rounded face;

2 those who want to look thinner and more defined; or

3 those who have strong features already, in which case contouring some areas is something to avoid.

If you're in the third category, you can have an early mark and move on to the next chapter! Those in the first two categories should read on. But first compare the 'before' shot at right with the finished look on page 39.

How to contour

Now remember, with contouring we're trying to create the illusion of a shadow, so we must use only matte colours with no shine or reflection, and also avoid any orange or red tones.

When applying shading, initially place the brush where you want the darkest shading to begin, as this is when you will have the most product on the brush. As you move the brush away from the starting point and along the contouring line, the amount of product will reduce and the shadow will fade. Keep a clean brush loaded with translucent powder or your shade of foundation on standby to help you blend.

Make sure you avoid any products with shine or reflection—the purpose of contouring is to create shadows, and it's not possible to do that with shiny/reflective products. Think matte greys, browns and taupes, even eye shadows.

Contouring is a powerful tool and a makeup artist's secret weapon but, like anything, it's only effective when used appropriately, so only apply it to places where it will have a positive effect.

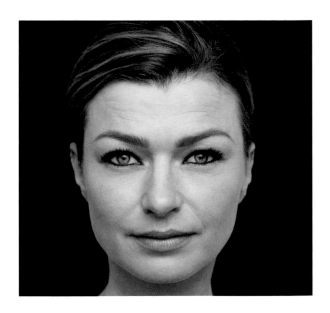

1 CHEEKBONES

In the following step-by-step photographs I used a cream foundation that's four shades darker than the model's skin tone. You can contour the cheekbones either before or after applying blush.

Step 1

Imagine drawing a line from the corner of your mouth to the top of your ear. You're creating a shadow that has the visual effect of pushing in the shaded area, so shading under this line will have the effect of lifting your cheekbone. The darkest part of the shading should be towards the ear, so start here and fade down into the cheek. To delicately define the feature, the shading should be no wider than your little finger—any wider and you'll create a hollowing effect in the shaded area. Repeat on the other side.

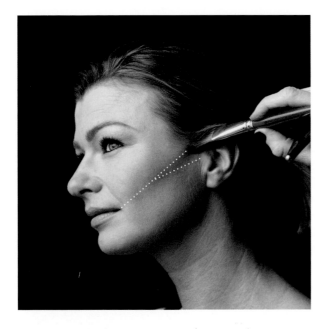

Always make sure you blend the edges of your shading thoroughly.

Step 2

This one is my favourite—it can take years off! Draw an imaginary line from the outer edge of your nose through the outer corner of your eye. This line should be parallel to the one you drew in step 1. Shading within the lines on the diagram will have the effect of indenting the temple, making the cheeks more prominent and also giving the eyes an incredible lift. Repeat on the other side.

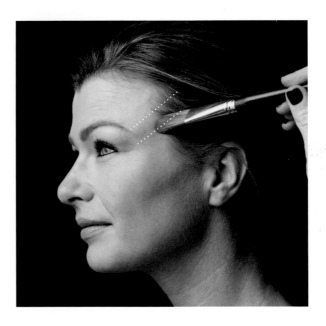

These two steps for contouring your cheekbones are great for:

• enhancing your cheekbones;

• thinning down a rounded face; and

• creating greater cheek definition.

However, they are unnecessary if:

• you're underweight;

• your cheekbones are already pronounced; or

• you have bony facial features.

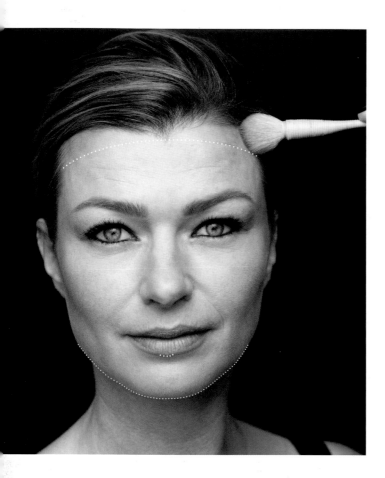

Shading the hairline is great for:

- a high forehead;
- softening a square, overly rounded or large forehead;
- helping to disguise a receding hairline; and
- a fine hairline (shading in this area reduces the visibility of the scalp so it can also reduce the appearance of thinning hair, but be careful if you're blonde, as contouring with shades of brown can be more obvious with lighter-coloured hair).

However, it is unnecessary if you have a:

- small forehead; or
- low hairline.

3 JAW LINE

The idea here is to define the jawbone, an area that cops a beating as you age. Creating your ideal jaw line may mean, depending on how it's holding up, applying the shading either under the jaw line or blending it onto your face to reduce the rather unattractive appearance of jowls. I also add strength and definition by always blending down the neck, starting dark at the jaw line.

Take a look in the mirror—if you have that very common white spot in the middle of your neck caused by lack of sun exposure, shade it too.

4 LIPS

Applying a tiny shadow under the bottom lip gives the illusion of a fuller bottom lip, while highlighting the upper lip will give you a fuller top lip (see page 73). This is a great technique if you have uneven lips.

2 HAIRLINE

If you have a large forehead, shading the hairline can have the effect of reducing its height, resulting in a more youthful face shape.

When shading this area, it's important to blend the colour into the hairline so that its edges completely disappear. Apply more shading in the temple areas and, as you move towards the middle of the forehead, taper the shading towards the hairline.

Use a kabuki brush or the contouring brush I've designed specially for this.

Makeup does not stop with your face—you must pay attention to your neck. Sometimes making the neck a shade or two darker than your face gives your jaw line and chin more definition, so don't be afraid to go one shade darker on your neck.

5 EYES

When shading the eyes, stay within the boundaries of the imaginary lines (as in the diagram) and follow the natural contour of the eye socket, although you can go slightly above the natural socket if your eyes are deep-set or showing signs of ageing. A brown matte shadow is perfect for this. Remember, you're doing this to contour and create shape, not create an eye shadow effect, so it should be undetectable and accentuate your facial features. Keep it soft.

If you don't have an obvious eye socket due to a droopy eyelid, apply the shading to the area you need to 'push back' in order to create the appearance of one (this is clearly demonstrated on Meme in Look 23, page 156).

For puffy eyelids, slightly darken the area below the brow so it will recede.

Shading the eyes is great for:

• defining eyes with a natural look;

• making smaller eyes look more open; and

• disguising puffy, hooded lids.

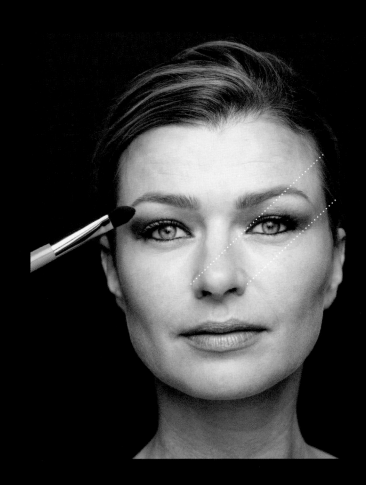

Blend, blend! Make sure you take the time to blend the shading well, and always check yourself carefully before you leave the house, especially your profile. You don't want to look as if you have unblended brown stripes all over your face—not a good look!

6 NOSE

If you're unhappy with your nose, you can use highlighter to shade it to the desired shape or width. Make sure you blend well, and take photos to make sure the effect is subtle, not obvious.

Depending on the problem, there are two techniques you can use.

1 If you don't like the shape of your nose, shade down its sides to define it or make it look straighter or smaller.

2 If you struggle to keep sunglasses on, chances are your nose bridge is a bit flat. Highlight the flat area in the centre of the bridge—see the dots between Jenny's eyes (opposite)—with a light concealer (the one you use under your eyes) or a soft, shimmery, skin-toned eye shadow that is lighter than your skin tone.

If your sunglassses never stop sliding off your nose, look for a pair designed specifically for this problem.

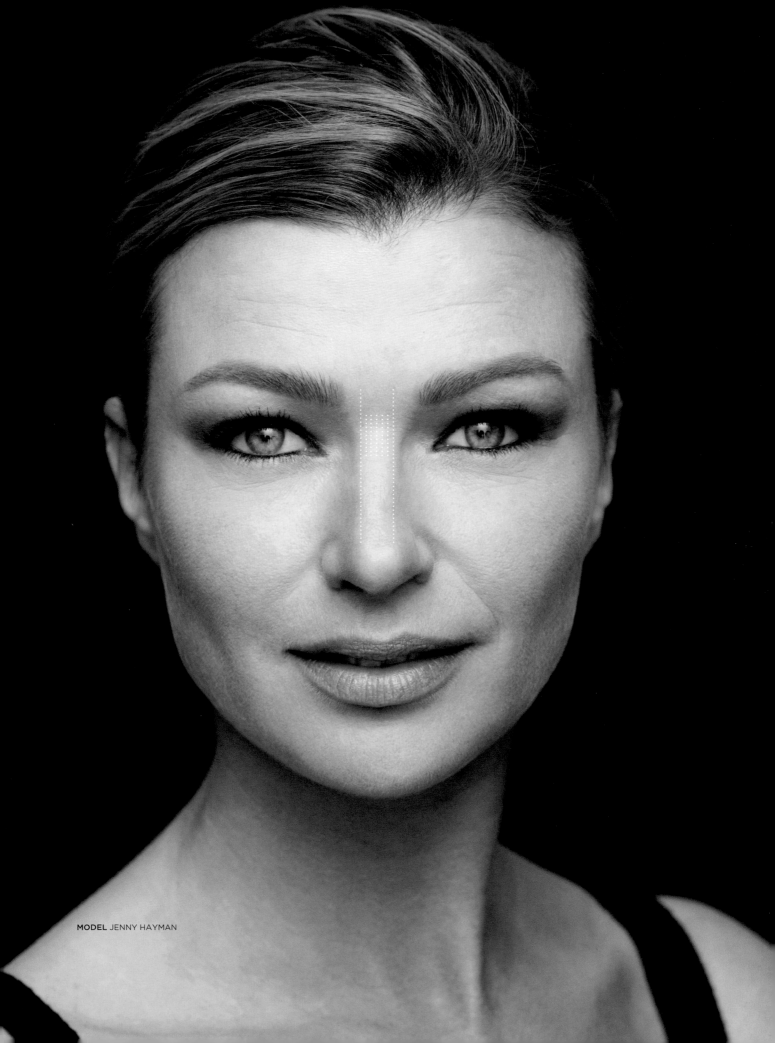

MODEL JENNY HAYMAN

Eyes

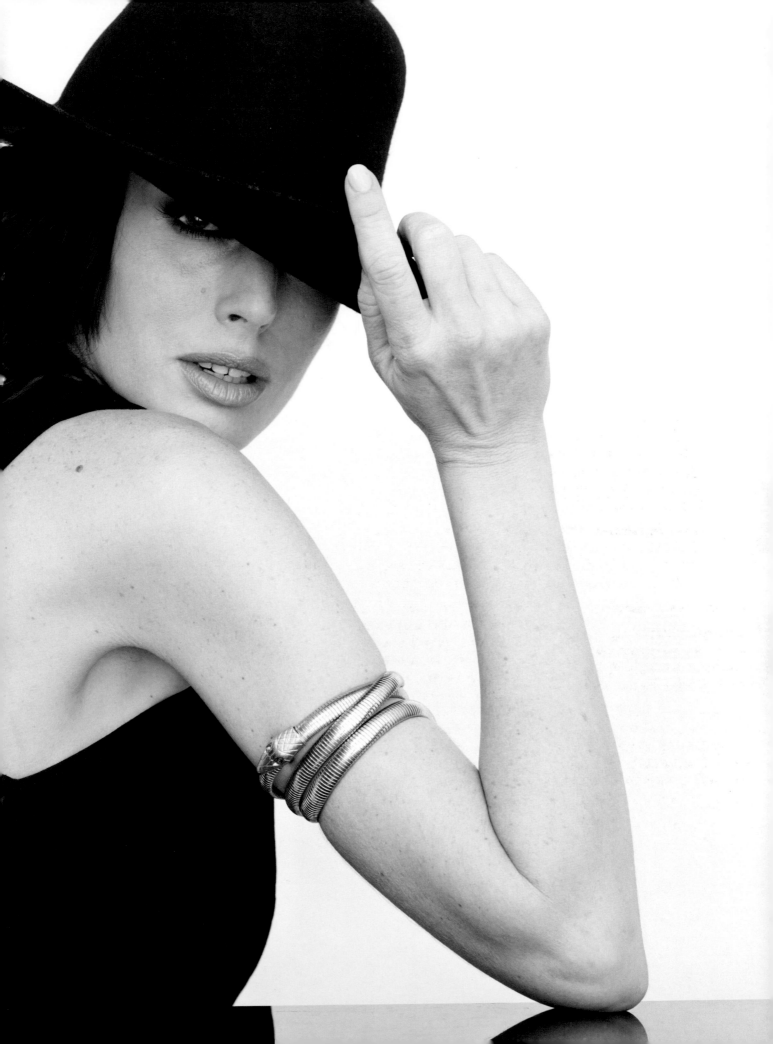

As you get older, the features around your eyes change. For example, as the eye socket deepens, it creates a protruding brow bone, which may make your eyes look hollow and sunken. Droopy eyelids can also develop, usually on the outer edge, creating a 'hooded' appearance. And then there's the hanging brow, which is like a second eyelid, but this one really means business!

The first rule is—don't panic. I have included lots of 'Looks' on pages 82–169 so you can see for yourself what a huge difference eye makeup can make when it's correctly applied. Simply find the model or celebrity with the look you're trying to achieve, or whose features are most like your own, and follow the steps to optimise your look.

Eyes first

Your eyes affect everything, including the overall shape of your face, so if you get your eye makeup right, you've pretty much nailed it. You'll notice that in a lot of the 'Looks' I do the eyes first. Most makeup books list foundation as the first step (and it sometimes is), but I believe the eyes are the most powerful feature of your face and you have to get them right before anything else.

There are two other reasons why I like to do the eyes first.

1 When you do your eyes, you often get constant eye shadow 'fallout' on your cheeks, which can ruin your foundation if you applied that first.

2 If you're going to run out of time when doing your makeup, do the most intricate or time-consuming part (your eyes) first. Applying foundation is quick and easy, and you can always do it in the car (as long as you're not the one driving, of course).

Remember, you must always prep your eyes—your eyelid is one of the oiliest parts of your face (see page 27). If you don't remove the oil, you can kiss your long-lasting eye shadow goodbye.

Most women don't know how to either enhance or minimise a certain eye shape. Regardless of your eye shape, my golden rule is to always extend eyeliners and eye shadows either one- or two-thirds of the way across the eye. If you only go halfway, you'll cut the eye in half and make it look distorted.

Take a look in the mirror and decide which of the following eye categories applies to you.

'SUNKEN EYES'

The most common eye issue for older women is 'sunken eyes'. If you have deep sockets with sunken eyes, rule number one is to lighten the deepest part of your eye lid (eye socket)—not darken it like most women do—and slightly darken anything that protrudes or looks puffy—for example, your brow bone. This will have the effect of 'raising' the socket. Never use shimmery shadows to do this, as they highlight wrinkles.

SMALL EYES

If you have small eyes, you can make them look larger. Simply curling your lashes and applying mascara, then applying creamy white, non-waterproof pencil to the inner rim will create the illusion of larger eyes. If you're feeling confident, you can enlarge the appearance of your eyes even more by adding single false lashes to the top outer lash line (see page 62).

LARGE OR PROTRUDING EYES

If you have very large, rounded or protruding eyes, never use hard-edged eyeliner, either above or below the eyes. If you do, it has the effect of 'framing' the eye, but in all the wrong ways, drawing more attention to both them and the saggy under-eye area. You can also make the shape more 'cat-like' by applying dark pencil to the inner rim of the eye, which helps to reduce the eye shape.

Keep dark colours to the outer third corner of the eye. Don't follow the natural shape of the eyes—try to make the outline of the eye shadow more rectangular, and extend it to the outer corner of the eye. Don't highlight the middle of the eyelid, and only apply mascara to the top lashes.

HEAVY EYELIDS

If you have heavy eyelids, apply eye shadow to the inner corners of your eyes, both the top and bottom, so you can still see the colour on your lids when your eyes are open. Make sure that your eyebrows aren't too arched, as this will accentuate heavy lids—go for a straighter brow shape with a slight arch. You can also use a matte contouring shade on the lids to give the illusion of a deeper-set socket.

CLOSE-SET EYES

For close-set eyes, use a highlighter in the inner corners to make them look as if they are further apart, and restrict all darkening, shading or 'smoking' to the outer corner of the eye—this means keeping false eye lashes on the outer corner as well. So the rule is—anything light, highlighting or metallic goes on the inner part of the eye, and anything dark or smoky goes on the outer part of the eye to 'wing' it out. Darkening the eye the whole way across will only accentuate close-set eyes.

SHORT EYELASHES

If you have very short eyelashes, get some lash extensions, or use false lashes. I use them all the time. See also the 'Lashes' section (page 62).

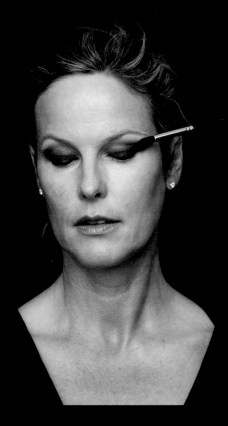

MODEL JENNY TAYLOR

Eye colour charts

The number one question people always ask me is: 'What colour suits me?' This is a very important question, as your eyes are the first facial feature people look at, followed by your lips. There are individual colours and colour families you can wear to enhance and harmonise your natural colouring and emphasise your best feature—your eyes!

When it comes to fashion, we often break the 'rules' to create a 'wow' factor or a dramatic visual effect. The first fashion checkpoint for me is always colour—before cut, fit, fabric or anything else. If you can get your colours right, you are more than halfway there.

So reading and using the eyecolour charts is one of the most important aspects of this book. Even if you perfectly colour match everything else, the wrong colour eye shadow can bring it all undone. The opposite is also true. If you have the wrong hair colour, clothing and/or accessories, the most magical lipstick in the universe won't be able to pull it all together.

Sometimes even I get confused about the difference between someone being 'warm/cool' or 'summer/winter', because it's based on a combination of your skin, eyes and hair, and all three aren't always the same tone—for example, you can have warm eyes with cool skin, or warm skin with cool hair.

Wearing the wrong colour around your eyes is worse than wearing the wrong-coloured shirt, so as a makeup artist I take this topic extremely seriously—so seriously that I consult with Bronwyn Fraser, an expert in colour science who knows more about colour than anyone else I know.

On the following pages I have revised and expanded the eye colour charts we introduced in *Makeup: The Ultimate Guide* to help you make your colour choices quickly and easily. The natural eye colours have been grouped into both warm and cool.

I've made these charts very easy for you to follow—simply locate your eye colour within one of the colour grids, and you'll find the perfect eye shadow colours for you.

The eye shadow charts are also divided into the following two groups:

1 colours that complement your natural eye colour; and

2 colours that intensify your natural eye colour and make it 'pop'.

The first chart (opposite) suits all eye colours, so I recommend you include two or three of these eye shadow colours in your makeup kit.

If you have green eyes, refer to the colour charts for green eyes on pages 50–1. On page 50 you'll find the perfect shades of green shadow to enhance or complement warm green eyes, while on page 51 are shades of violet that will intensify cool green eyes. Because violet is opposite to green on the colour wheel, using violet shades will make your eyes look greener than they've ever looked before.

All the shades in the charts can also be used in eyeliners, pencils or highlighters, but remember, always stick to matte shades, as metallics enhance any wrinkles you may have.

Refer to these colour charts whenever you go shopping for makeup—you will feel much more confident about the colours that actually suit you and you'll also be able to say 'no' to the 'colour of the season', 'cos it ain't in season if it ain't your colour!

All eye colours

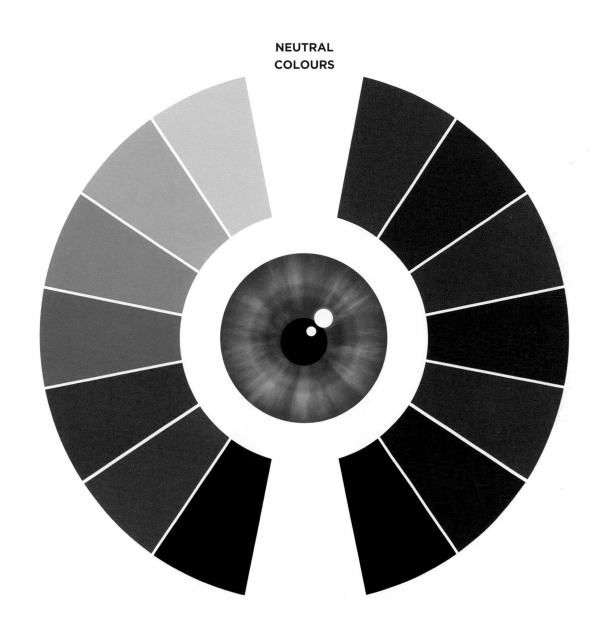

NEUTRAL COLOURS

Blue eyes

Warm blue

COMPLEMENTARY COLOURS   OR   **INTENSIFYING COLOURS**

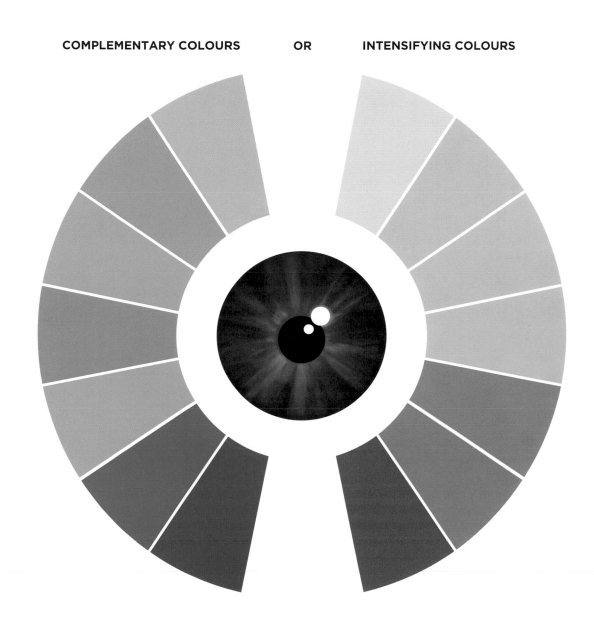

Cool blue

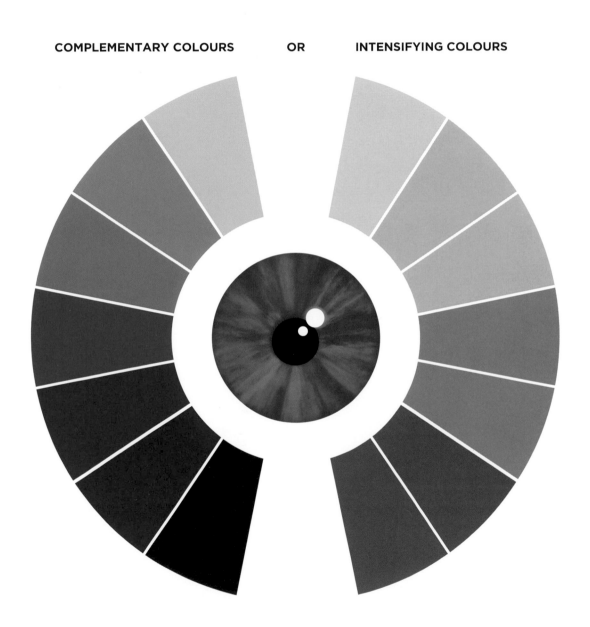

Brown eyes

Warm brown

COMPLEMENTARY COLOURS　　　OR　　　**INTENSIFYING COLOURS**

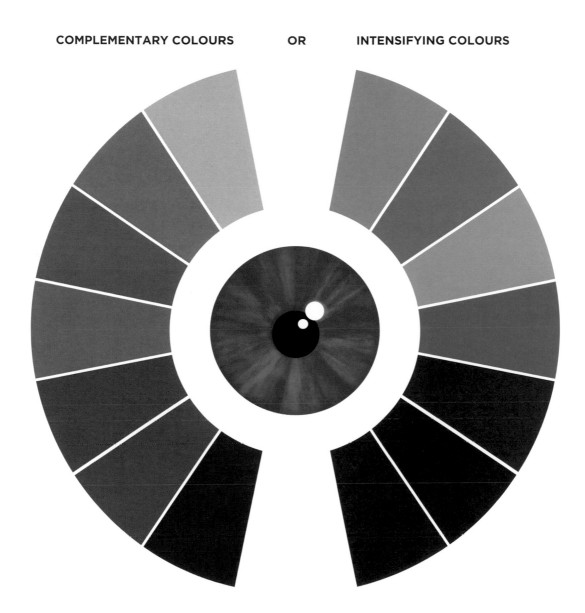

Cool brown

COMPLEMENTARY COLOURS   OR   INTENSIFYING COLOURS

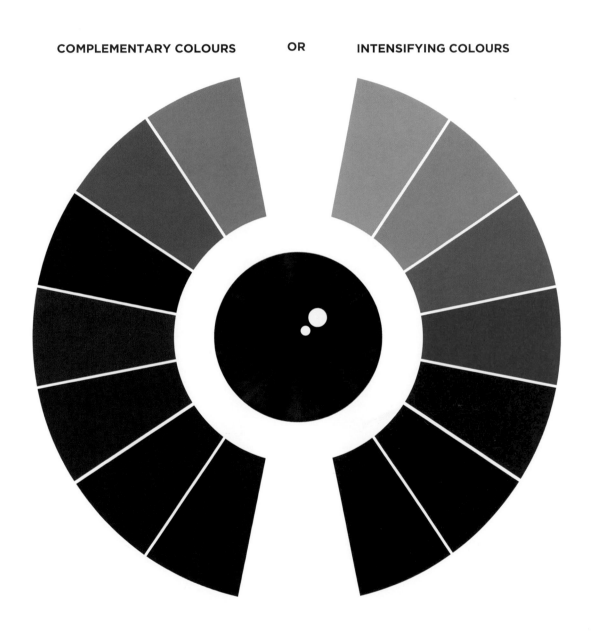

Green eyes

Warm green

COMPLEMENTARY COLOURS   **OR**   **INTENSIFYING COLOURS**

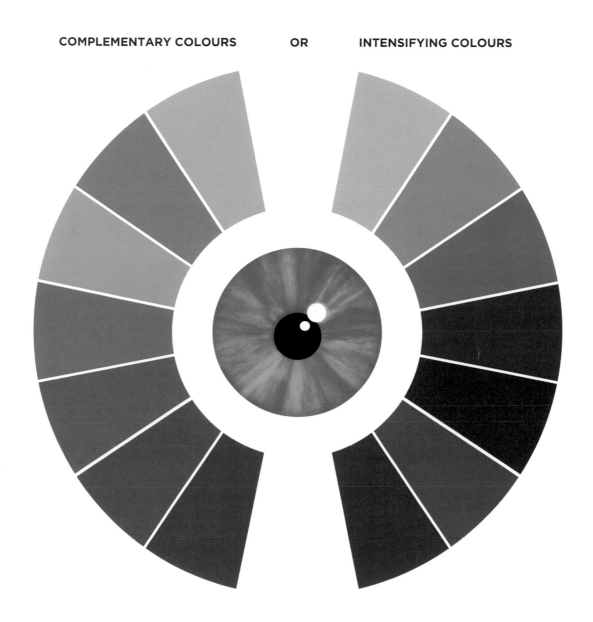

Cool green

COMPLEMENTARY COLOURS   **OR**   **INTENSIFYING COLOURS**

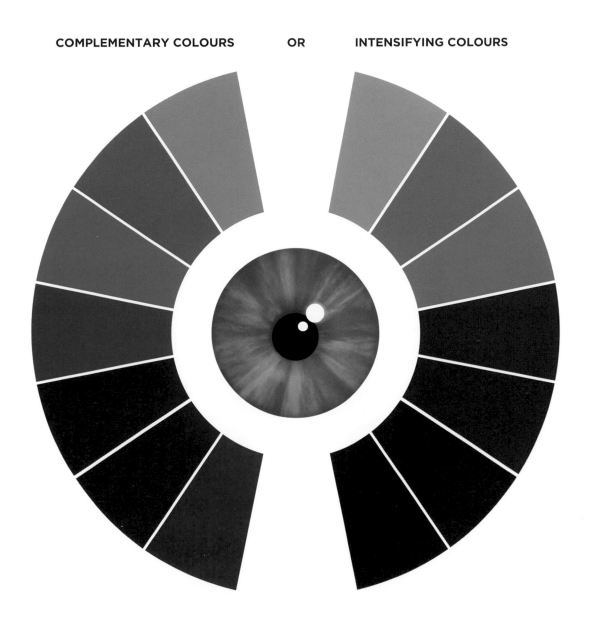

Hazel eyes

True hazel

COMPLEMENTARY COLOURS   **OR**   **INTENSIFYING COLOURS**

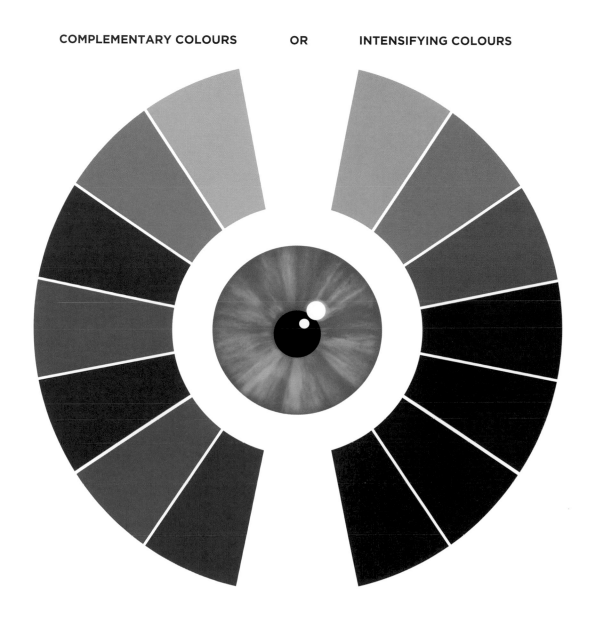

Golden hazel

COMPLEMENTARY COLOURS   OR   **INTENSIFYING COLOURS**

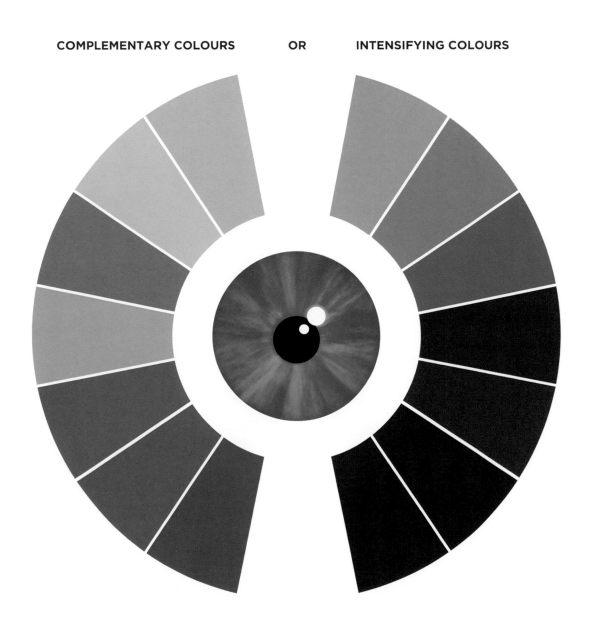

Eyebrows

Getting your eyebrows right gives you a fantastic foundation for the rest of your face, especially your eyes. If you've read any of my earlier books, such as *Makeup: The Ultimate Guide*, you'll know that eyebrows get me onto my soapbox! Don't worry, I'll show you how to achieve the perfect brow, but this time I'm going to approach it from a different angle, by asking—what can your eyebrows do for you?

Your Mum's advice was to arch your brows, to lift your eyes as you age, but this is probably one of the worst things you can do—your eyebrows should not be part of your hairline!

Your eyebrows do change as you get older—the hairs can become sparser and grey hairs emerge. These and other changes mean that the shape that worked for you when you were younger needs to be adapted to suit the changes around your eyes. The good news is that your eyebrows, when done correctly, can play a major role in reducing the signs of ageing.

But what if you have no eyebrows left? There are some male hair restoration products designed for hereditary baldness on the market that work effectively in restoring brow hair (as long as it was there in the first place). But even without this, you can effectively shape your brow line with the correct use of a brow pencil (we'll cover this when we create the perfect brow—see page 56).

One of the most prominent signs of getting older is sunken eyes, which make your brow bone look as if it's protruding. So the last thing you want to do is arch your brows and give the impression that it protrudes even more. The perfect brow should cut right through the brow bone, lowering the arch and decreasing its prominence (see the following pages).

Achieving the perfect brow can do some amazing things, such as dramatically narrow and straighten your nose; reduce the prominence of puffy eyelids (which will take off ten years as well as five kilograms!); and lift your eyes.

EYEBROW EXCESSES

When you were younger, you could probably do everything in excess and get away with most of it. But once you're over 40, you're told to do everything in moderation—no more excess. This is equally true of eyebrows. If you avoid the three eyebrow excesses listed below, you will literally take years off your face.

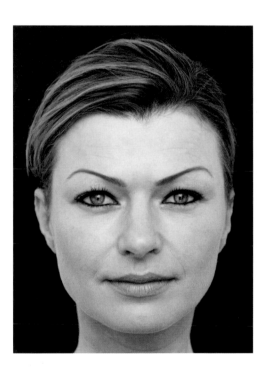

1 EXCESSIVE LIFT

If you lift or arch the brow dead centre, the resultant downhill slant on the outer edge will create a huge, saggy, puffy eyelid that will age you considerably. Remember, what goes up, must come down...and you never want to come down on the outer edge of your eyes.

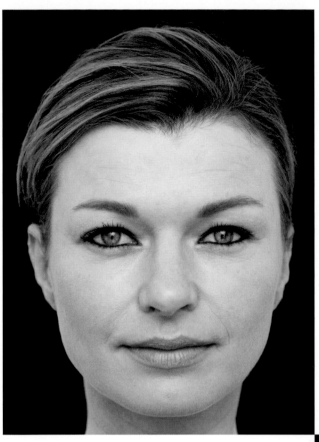

2 EXCESSIVE GAP

The further apart your eyebrows are, the wider your nose will look. As you age, your nose does tend to get a bit bigger, so the last thing you want to do is draw attention to it.

3 EXCESSIVE ROUNDING

Do not use a protractor to trace your eyebrows, as it will make your eyebrows look like the letter 'M'. Unless you want a 'drive thru' look, this is not a good thing, as it creates too much space between your lash line and your brows, accentuating the deepset inner corners of your eyes and any shadows underneath. It also immediately adds years to your face by making your eyes look puffy and droopy. If you have saggy, heavy lids, this is the worst shape. You can only get away with this if you have very flat lids, but why risk it?

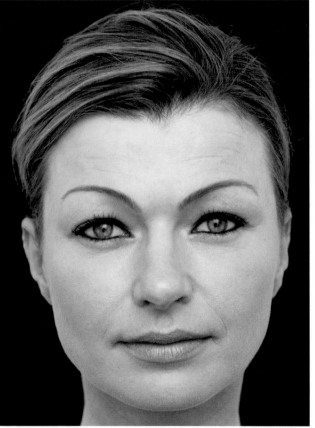

THE EYEBROW ARSENAL

To sculpt and maintain the perfect brow, you need a few essential items in your makeup kit that will make all the difference. If you've only just realised that your brows are all out of whack, it will take time to groom them back into shape. Trust me, it's worth the effort.

- **Brow mascara** A great tool for temporarily lightening or darkening your eyebrows, this product is hard to find, so you may need to buy it from a specialist makeup outlet.

- **Brow pencil** Make sure your brow pencil matches your brow colour exactly. You can use your pencil to subtly change (or emphasise) your brow shape, and you'll be amazed at the difference it can make.

- **Brow shadow** As with the brow pencil, simply apply this with an angled brush.

- **Tweezers** A good pair of tweezers is essential for initially sculpting and then maintaining the perfectly shaped brow.

- **Eyebrow tinting** You might want to consider having your eyebrows tinted when getting your hair professionally coloured, but please make sure the hairdresser matches or complements your hair colour!

THE PERFECT BROW

The perfect brow narrows and straightens your nose and lifts your eyes. The less you arch your brows, the younger you'll look. If you've got it wrong until now, you're in for an instant facelift!

If you've gone nuts with your tweezers in the past, as of now declare your brows an environmental protection zone and use the brow pencil as your guide for selective regrowth. Draw your ideal shape and don't pluck any hairs that fall within it. Over time your natural brows may return and you'll be able to reduce your pencil artwork.

As you read the following guide to achieving the perfect brow, refer to the photograph on the opposite page.

- **Nose bridge line** The gap between your brows should match the width of your *ideal* nose bridge. This creates the illusion of a thinner, more refined nose.

- **Brow starting point (inner)** Always start with a right angle, as this will give you an immediate eyelift. If your brows don't come in this far, use a brow pencil to draw it in—this can serve as a guide for which hairs not to remove in the future.

- **Brow arch point** The top of your eyebrow arch should be two-thirds of the way across your brow and in line with the outer edge of your iris. But remember, there should be no excessive lift. As you age, your lids become fuller and puffier, so lowering the arch creates a more youthful appearance.

- **Brow end point (outer)** Imagine a line from the bottom edge of your nose to the outer corner of your eye and beyond. The brow should at least touch that line, but if it falls short, your eyes will look a bit distorted and your brows will appear too masculine and severe. If your brows don't extend far enough to reach the guideline, use a brow pencil to bridge the gap. If you overdo it, dip an angled brush in your foundation and use it as an eraser to create the perfect end point.

- **Grooming** Once you have the brow shape sorted, apply hair lacquer to a clean mascara wand and comb up and out. This will maintain the starting point at a right angle and lengthen the end point so it's in line with the end point guideline—it'll give you an instant eyelift.

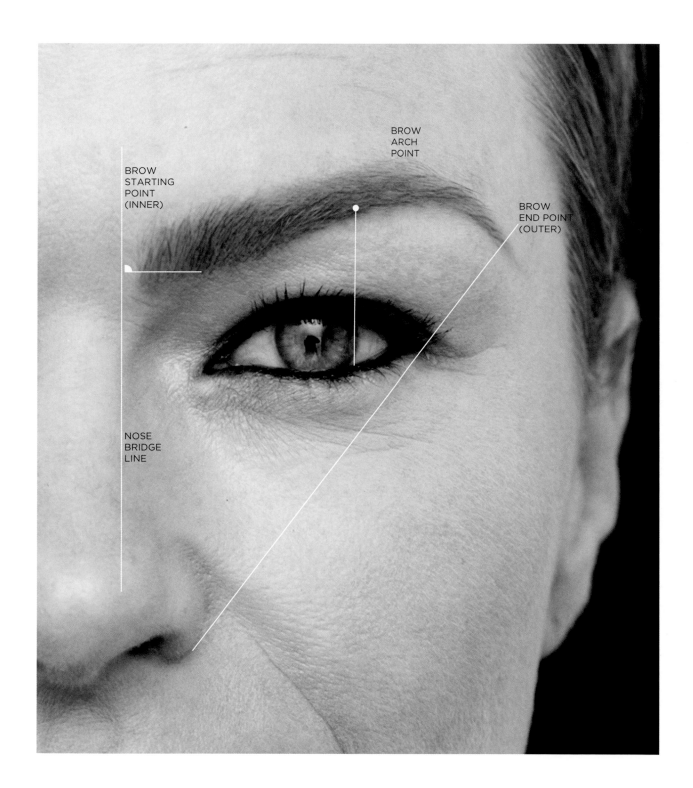

BROW
STARTING
POINT
(INNER)

BROW
ARCH
POINT

BROW
END POINT
(OUTER)

NOSE
BRIDGE
LINE

HOW TO SHAPE THE PERFECT BROW #1

You can see how over-arching the brow creates an instant puffy eyelid while the wide space between the brows accentuates the hollowness in the inner corners. Lowering her brows makes Jenny look more youthful.

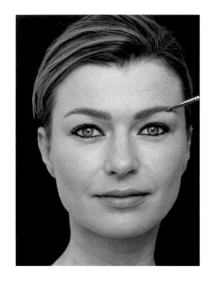

2 PLUCK YOUR BROWS

In the best light possible, use pointed tweezers to pluck unwanted brow hairs and help create that sharp right angle.

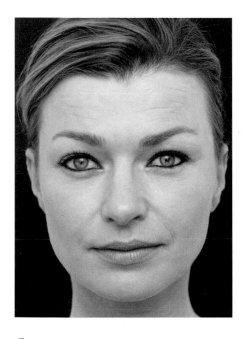

1 PREP YOUR SKIN

Prep your skin, then apply a water-based primer or moisturiser.

If there are areas in your brows that are less dense than others, use a brow pencil to fill in the gaps, but don't trace the entire brow. This way you get the shape while maintaining a natural look.

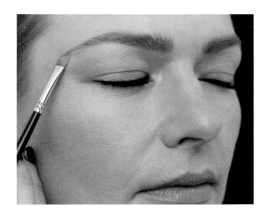

3 TAPER THE LINE

To make a perfect clean end, take a clean, fine angled brush with a hint of foundation and wipe underneath the line.

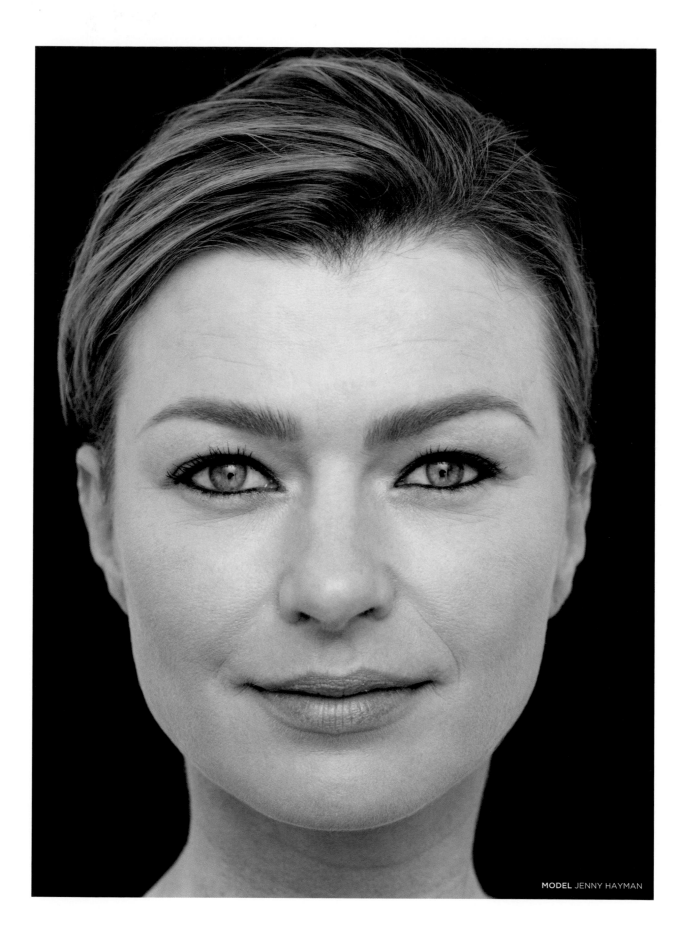

MODEL JENNY HAYMAN

HOW TO SHAPE THE PERFECT BROW #2

In the first shot you can see how having her brows so far apart accentuates the hollowness at the inner corners of Olga's eyes.

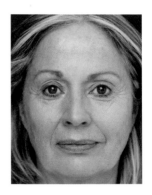

1 PREP YOUR SKIN

Prep your skin, then apply a water-based primer or moisturiser.

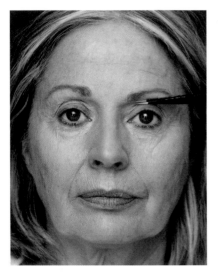

2 PLUCK YOUR BROWS

In the best light possible, use pointed tweezers to pluck unwanted brow hairs and help create that sharp right angle.

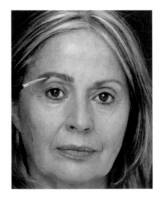

3 APPLY FINE LINES

Use a perfectly matched brow shadow and a fine angled brush to apply fine strokes at the angle you want the hairs to sit— vertical in the centre but at an angle towards the outer brow.

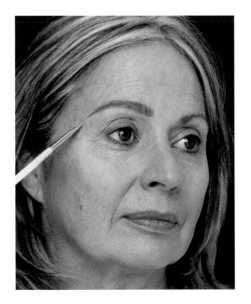

4 TAPER THE LINE

To make a perfect clean end, take a clean, fine angled brush with a hint of foundation and wipe underneath the line.

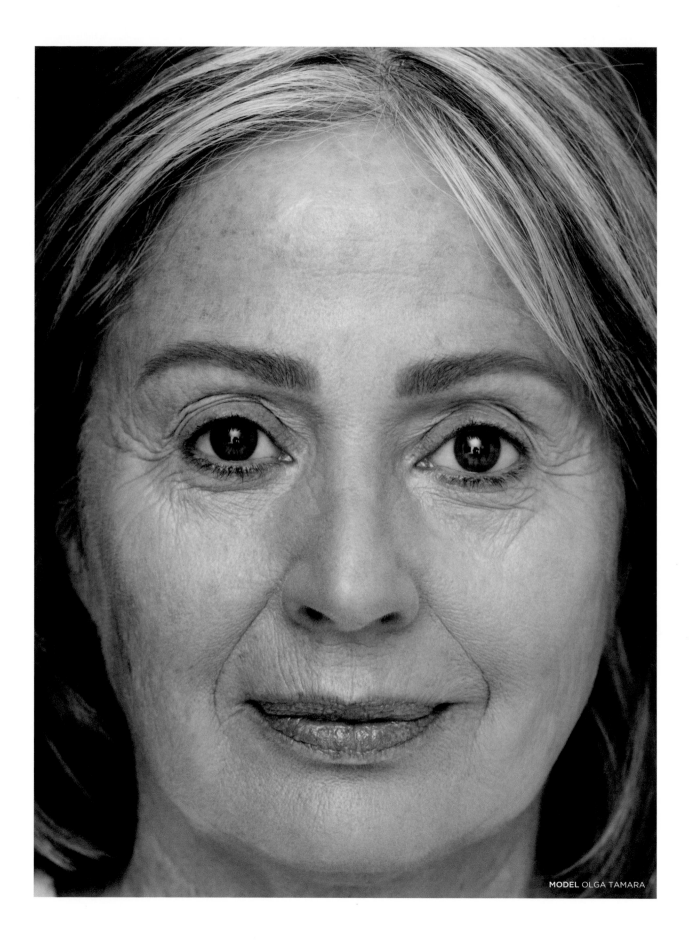

MODEL OLGA TAMARA

Lashes

I have deliberately left the word 'false' out of this heading, as that's the last thing your lashes should look like. But as you age, your eyelashes do become depleted, and a false lash can make all the difference, highlighting your best asset—your eyes!

I know the idea of applying false lashes can be daunting if you haven't done it before, but with the right tools and just a few minutes, nothing will enhance your eyes like a set of great lashes. And there's more! With false lashes you will never have runny mascara again, so you will be able to 'tear up' without suffering the consequences.

The first rule of false lashes is to always apply them with latex (lash glue). While most lashes come with a small tube, it is best to use duo latex, which you can find in most makeup stores. But whatever type of latex you use, make sure it's waterproof, otherwise tears, rain or an unplanned swim will leave you looking 'interesting'.

The second rule is to use an eyelash applicator. I honestly don't know how I ever applied lashes without them.

When it comes to the lashes themselves, the base of the lash—that is, the seam on which they are sewn—will be either clear or black. If it's clear, they will look more natural and blend with your own lashes. If the base is black, you'll get an eyeliner effect on your eyelids, which can be great, depending on the look you're going for.

If you want the effect of false lashes, but can't see well enough to apply them, try lash extensions. They'll last for 6–8 weeks and you won't have to use mascara.

TYPES OF LASHES

To achieve an ageless, classic look, choose from these three lash types.

- **Individual lashes** When using single top lashes, apply them mostly to the outer corners, as this lifts the eyes and gives them a sexy look.

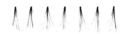

- **3/4 wispy lash** This lash is soft and wispy on the ends, with a clear base, which results in a natural look. If you've never used false eyelashes before, this is a great lash to start with—it's easy to apply and looks fabulous.

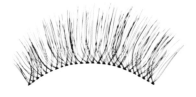

- **3/4 lash** This is the type I use the most. It fits every eyelid and is easy to apply. While the base of this lash is black (so you get the eyeliner effect), it only extends three-quarters of the way across your eyelid, so you'll have to extend your eyeliner the rest of the way.

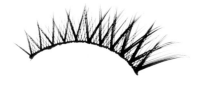

HOW TO APPLY FALSE LASHES

It's easy to find good lashes—they're sold every-where, from department stores to pharmacies. I constantly recommend 'new finds' on my YouTube channel, 'raemorrismakeup'.

Make sure you don't have your first go at applying false lashes just before a big night out. That's a sure-fire recipe for complete panic and ongoing social anxiety! Practise first!

Follow the instructions on page 64, then check out the photographs on the following pages to see how using different types of lashes can completely change your overall look. All the lashes have been cut to 3/4 size, as the short lashes blend in so well with the natural ones.

To remove lashes, simply use warm water on a cotton pad. Hold the cotton pad over your eye for about two minutes, and the latex should easily fall away. In most cases you'll be able to reuse the lashes.

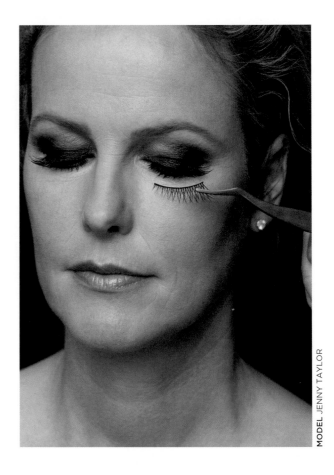

MODEL JENNY TAYLOR

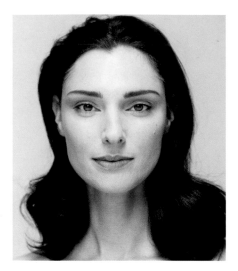

1 NATURAL LASHES

Check that your natural lashes are no longer than the false lashes you're going to apply.

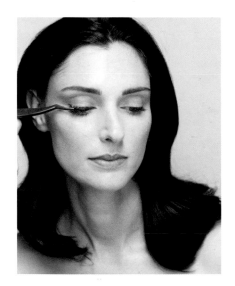

2 APPLY THE FALSE LASHES

Most lashes are too long, so you might need to trim the outer corner. Apply eyelash glue to the inner rim of the fake lashes, then wait until the glue is tacky before applying them. It's important to stretch your eyelid, then look down and sideways when you apply, starting on the outer corner of each eye. Make sure the fake lashes are on your natural lashes, not on the skin of your eyelid. I am applying false lashes only to Anneliese's top lashes, as it's a nightmare to apply them to the bottom ones.

3 USE THE APPLICATOR

Once the false lashes are in place and secure, use the eyelash applicator to pinch the false and natural lashes together. This will give your lashes a natural look.

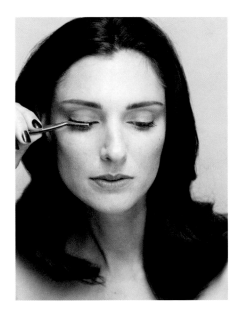

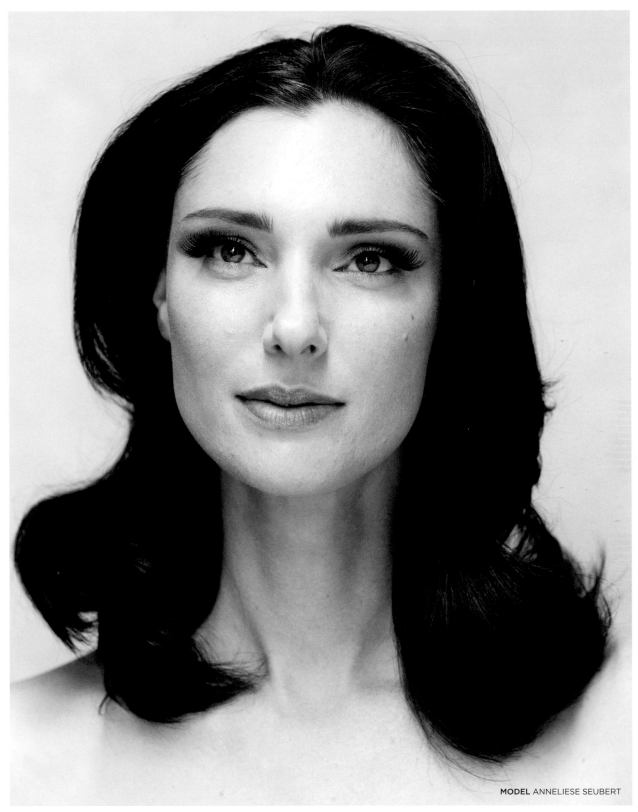

MODEL ANNELIESE SEUBERT

THE 3/4 LASH—THE MOST DRAMATIC, AND VERY SCREEN SIREN. PERFECT FOR A COCKTAIL PARTY.

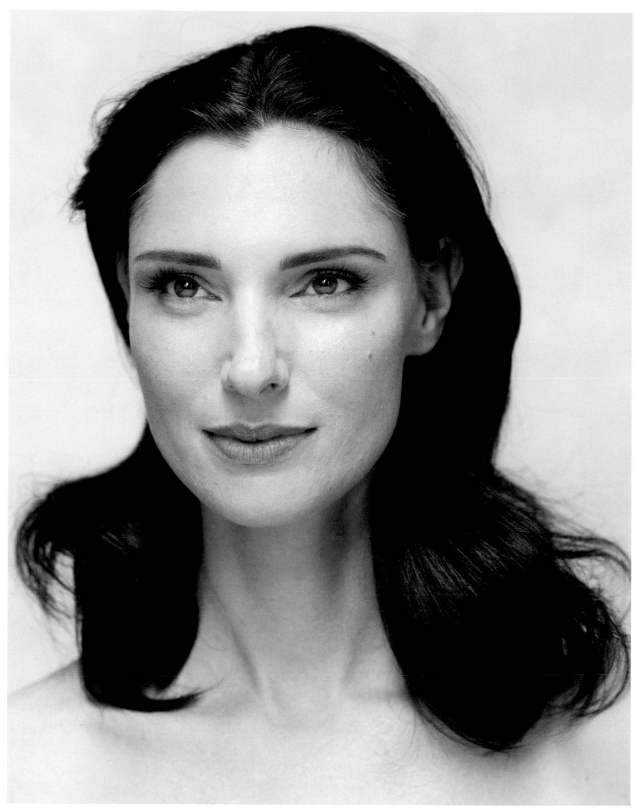

INDIVIDUAL LASHES GIVE YOU A VERY FRESH, HEALTHY LOOK.

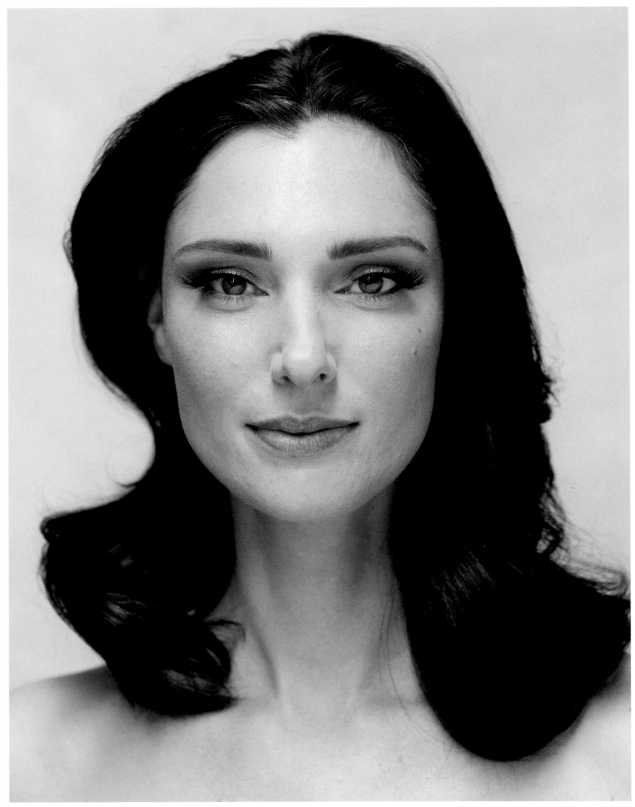

THE 3/4 WISPY LASH IS PERFECT FOR DAY.

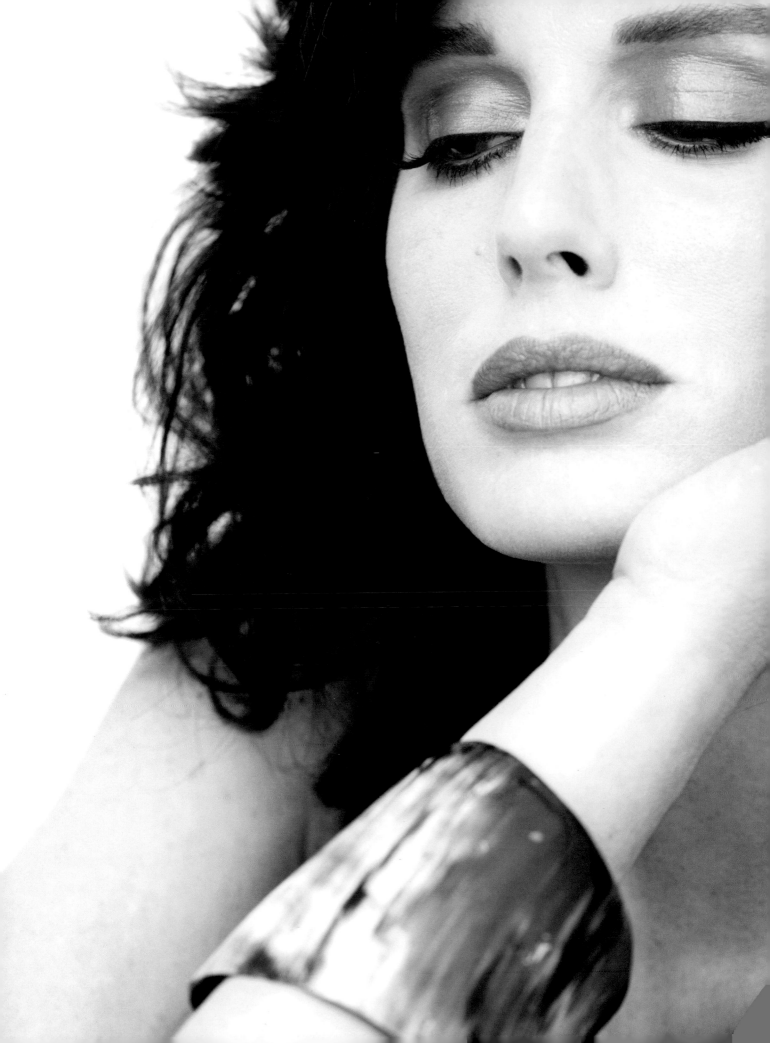

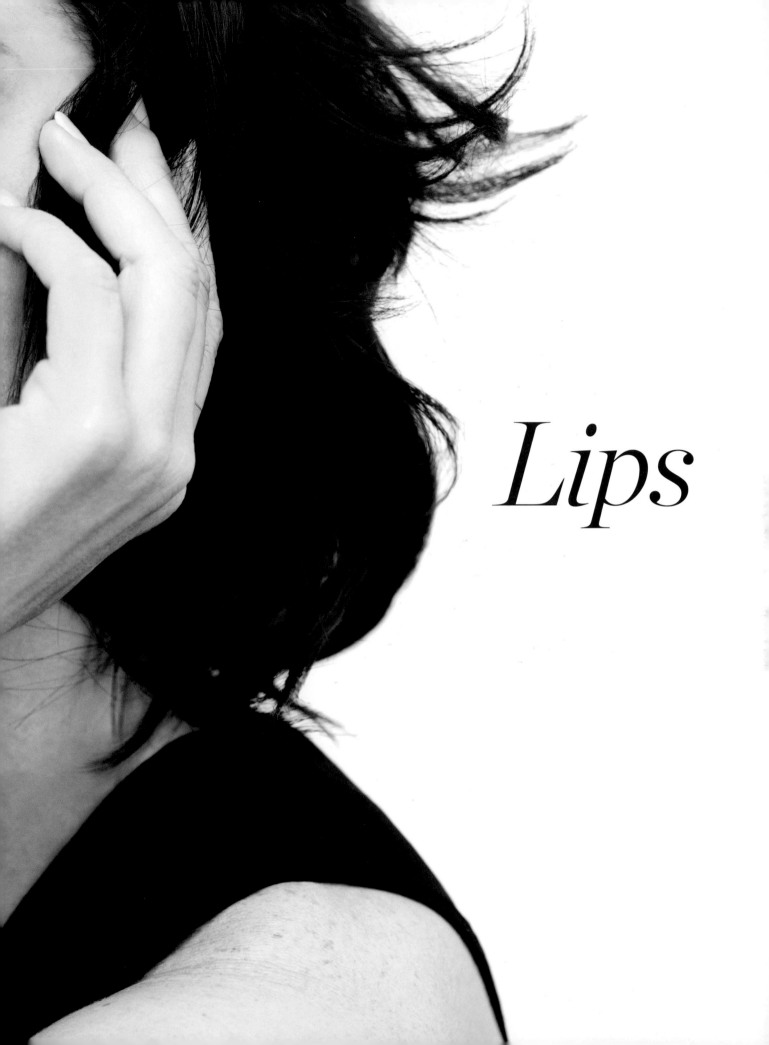

Lips

Your lips are one of your most powerful facial assets. Unfortunately, they are also one of the key signs of ageing on your face, so how you do your lips will have a huge impact on how old you look.

A myth handed down from our mothers is that the older we get, the more colour we need. I agree with this completely, but it's where you put the colour that makes all the difference. If you have plump, youthful lips (or close to whatever you had when you were 18), go for my favourite strong lip colours—brick red, rich burgundy and deep plums. These suit all women and are, in my opinion, the most elegant.

But if you're showing some signs of ageing, see the step-by-step instructions on page 73.

Choosing the right lipstick

Next time you're at the cosmetics counter, watch how most women choose their lipstick—by rubbing it backwards and forwards on the back of their hand until they find the shade they're after.

But your lip and the back of your hand couldn't be more different—lips have a blue-red tone, whereas the skin on the back of most hands is nude/neutral—so this isn't a reliable test. Instead, use the tip of your finger, which is close to both the texture and colour of your lips. You should be able to find the shade you want with one stroke of lipstick across the top of your finger. If it doesn't look good, pick another shade.

This trick will not only make your lipstick easier to apply, it will also save you a lot of money, as you won't need to use half your lipstick to achieve the colour you want. If you apply lipstick with only one stroke, it won't bleed or melt, and if the colour is too strong, it's easy to soften it.

Choosing the right shade

We have to distinguish here between 'nude' (that is, natural) and 'dead', because if your lips end up paler than your skin tone, that's what you'll look like—dead.

Some women need lip colour, and others don't. To find out which category you fall into, follow these steps.

1 With no makeup on, pull your hair back from your face.

2 Nude down your lips with foundation.

If you look ill, it will only be possible for you to wear this look if you have gone for dramatic eye makeup. If your eyes come alive, you pass, and can successfully wear a nude lip!

Five golden rules

Here are my golden rules for perfect lips.

1 LIP SHADE

As with wardrobe and eyeshadow colours, most people fall into one of two colour categories for lipstick—cool or warm.

Here's an easy way to find out whether you fall into the 'cool' or 'warm' category. Scrape your hair back from your face, which should be free of any makeup, and try on two T-shirts—one should be pink for cool and the other orange for warm.

If you look good in the pink T-shirt, not the orange one, you should always look for cool or mahogany/pink undertone lipstick shades, cool reds (think wine shades), all pink shades, pink-based nudes and pink-based browns. Steer clear of anything with orange or warm brown.

On the other hand, if you picked orange, you probably go for gold jewellery, earthy clothing colours, orange, caramels, creams as opposed to whites, and so on. You should go for lipsticks in orange, corals, brick reds, warm browns, peachy nudes, all bronze shades—in short, anything warm. You can even highlight with a dash of gold!

If you're stuck, go for anything in a wine shade, such as mahogany or plum. These are the only colours in the colour spectrum that are both cool and warm, and they suit everyone because these are the colours we were all born with. Any skin colour, any age will suit these colours, which is why, if you look closely, you'll see so much of it on women walking the red carpet.

Watch for the contrasting effect your lip shade has on the appearance of your teeth. Cool-coloured lip shades (cool reds, all pinks and wine colours) will make your teeth look whiter, whereas brown shades can make your teeth look slightly yellow.

2 LIP LINER
Never use a lip liner that's a completely different colour to your lipstick. If you're using a lip liner, pencil in the whole lip so that, if your lipstick fades, you're not left looking like Bobo the clown.

3 LIP GLOSS
If your lips are naturally lined or wrinkled, don't overuse lip gloss. If you do, we're not talking about a lipstick bleed here, we're talking haemorrhage! Instead, go for velvety or more matte-textured lipsticks, and apply just a little gloss to the very centre of your lips.

4 LIP HAIR
Bleaching just doesn't cut it, as any lip hair, even if it is blond, will grow down to the lip line, making it impossible to create a sharp edge.

I prefer to use a hair-removing machine which, unlike waxing, doesn't remove any skin. I don't recommend hair-removal creams, as I don't believe a product that removes and dissolves 'hard keratin' (protein), such as hair, can do so without affecting the more sensitive 'soft keratin' (skin) underneath.

5 FOUNDATION
Don't apply foundation to your lips and then lipstick over the top of it. It's fine to use foundation on your lips to create a nude effect, but it doesn't work under lipstick—you just end up with a cakey white line all around your lips. This is because foundation and lipstick are often made of incompatible components—for example, water and grease—so they don't blend together. If you want a nude look, go for a nude lipstick shade.

Dry lips

As you age, your lips tend to become drier but, believe it or not, you can exfoliate them and achieve a plumper, more youthful look.

1 First, load up your lips with clear lanolin, the pure version. This is also sold as 'nipple cream', which is super safe—I mean, if a baby can cope with it, it must be OK! Don't use white lanolin or you'll look as if you belong on a cricket pitch—and zinc will never be in fashion!

2 Soothe some moisturiser into your lips to soften the dead skin, which will make it easier to remove.

3 Next, mix some bicarbonate of soda with a water-based cleanser and gently scrub your lips (see also 'Face and body scrub', page 11).

4 Finally, reapply the lanolin and allow it to soak into your lips while you do your makeup, then remove any excess.

5 Apply your lip colour.

If you're planning on using a matte shade, there's no need to moisturise beforehand, as you can always apply a little afterwards if your lips are too dry—matte lipstick can dry out your lips and make them look like cracked mud, which only emphasises any lines.

How to apply lipstick

If your lips have started to show signs of ageing, follow the instructions opposite each time you apply lipstick. I haven't extended the lip colour to the outer corners (which is where your lips start to age and droop). Remember, soft rose shades—the colours of youth—will give the illusion of bigger lips. This is because you avoid having a definitive border and what can potentially be an unflattering lip shape.

Nude lips look fuller because there is no defined border.

One trick I use throughout this book is to highlight the cupid's bow on the upper lip with some form of shimmer, which makes lips look fuller. This is much more effective than using a lip liner, which is severe and unflattering.

If you only use one stroke to apply your lipstick, you minimise the chances of it running.

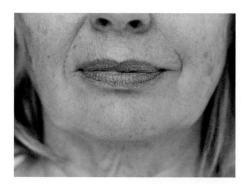

1 FOUNDATION AND POWDER

After applying foundation to your face and completing your makeup, lightly apply translucent powder around your lip line. This will help prevent any lip bleeds.

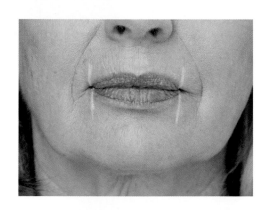

2 OUTER LIMITS

These vertical lines show the outer limits of where your lipstick should be taken—any further and you'll accentuate the downward angle of the lip corners.

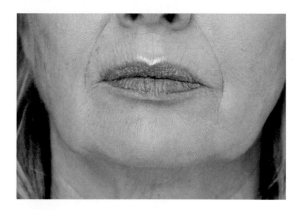

3 CUPID'S BOW

Apply shimmer to the cupid's bow.

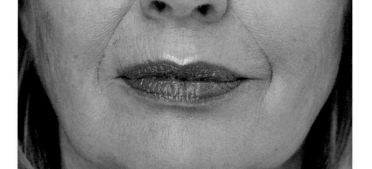

4 LIPSTICK

Apply lipstick.

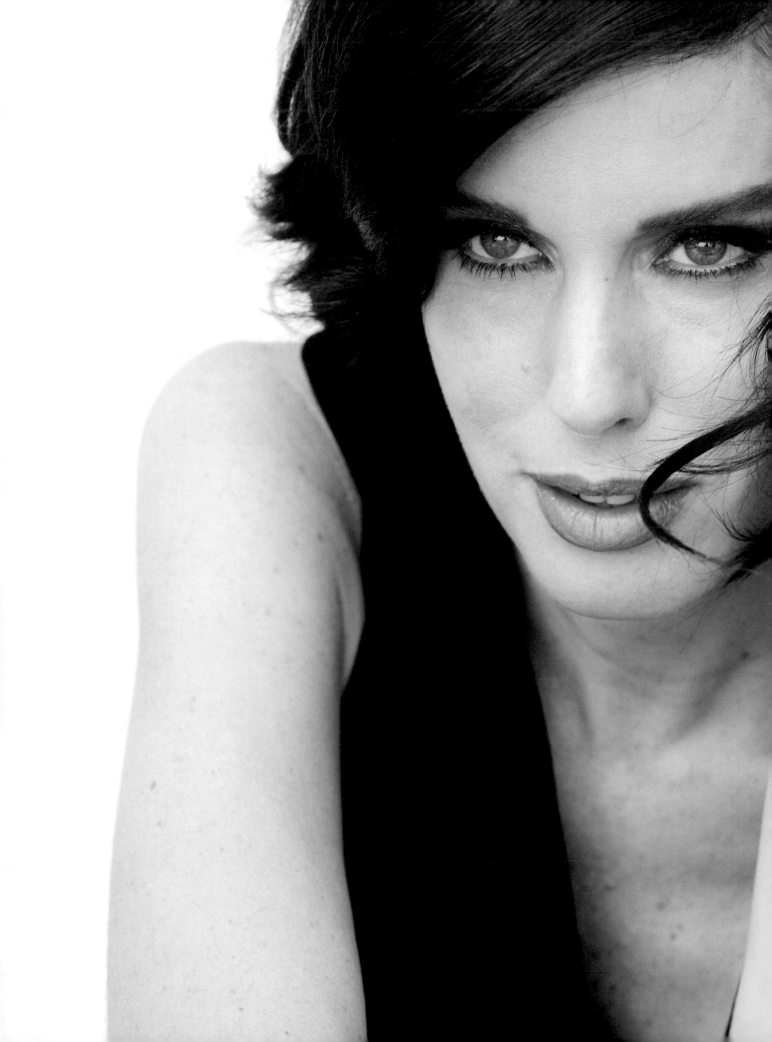

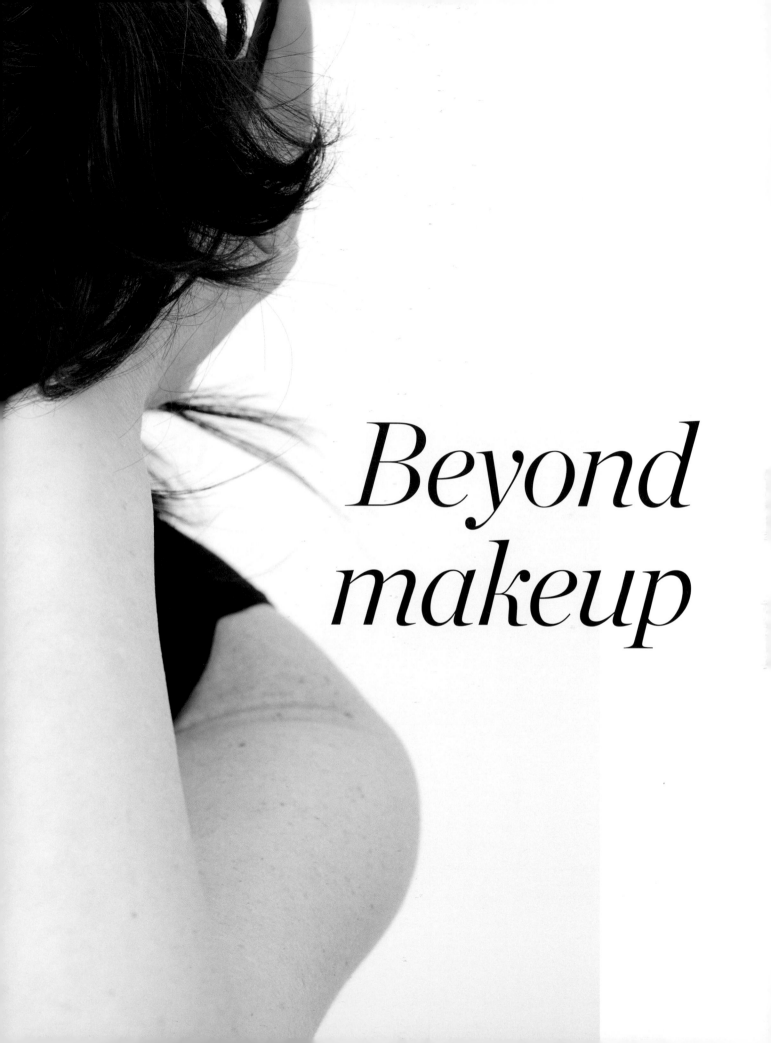

Beyond
makeup

It's not just your makeup that determines how you look—your clothing, hair and the environment (either indoors or outdoors) all affect your appearance. Have you ever been to a wedding or other special occasion thinking you look absolutely fabulous, only to see the photos a few weeks later and think, 'What the...?'

Here are some killer tips that will maximise the work you've put into your look.

The importance of lighting

One of the golden rules of photographing people is—light from below (up-light) is amazing, light from above (down-light) is bad. Down-light results in massive shadows on all the parts of your face that accentuate ageing, especially under your eyes. Up-light has the opposite effect—brightening, softening and lifting. So extending this theme, how do we apply it in practical terms?

- Always up-light—up, up, up! For example, for a dinner party at home, set the table with shiny white tablecloths and candles—anything that reflects onto your face from below.

- Try to avoid having your photo taken outside between 10 am and 2 pm—the lighting is just all wrong (think of the sun as the biggest down-light in the universe!). Even supermodels refuse to be shot outside at this time of day.

- If you don't have a choice about being photographed in the middle of the day—perhaps you're being snapped at a work do—insist that the person holding the camera turns on the flash.

- Using the flash has the same effect as an up-light, blowing out any dark shadows and skin imperfections, and flattening out bumps and hollows—like using a soft filter on the camera.

- Always ask the person taking the photograph to hold the camera above your eye line, as anything lower will make your jaw and neck look bigger.

- If you're feeling tired, wear a white shirt, which will reflect light onto your face—a great tip from fashion designer Peter Morrissey.

Clothes

Create and express your own timeless personal style in the way you dress and accessorise. If you're a slave to fashion, you might end up looking older than you really are.

- Wear colours that complement your skin tone and hair colour. (To find out whether you fall into the 'warm' or 'cool' category, see page 70.)

- Use dark colours to disguise any figure faults, such as a thick waist.

- Wear well-fitted garments, neither too tight nor too loose, and buy underwear that helps sculpt your body—my favourites are Trinny and Susannah's Original Magic Knickers, available from trinnyandsusannah.com.

- Invest in a simple little black dress that comes to just above the knee—a must-have for every stylish woman!

- If you have great legs, go for skirts and dresses that stop just above the knee, but avoid minis.

- Add style to your outfit with disinctive shoes and sleek stockings.

- Disguise an ageing neck and décolletage with a scarf.

- Hide droopy earlobes with a pair of fabulous light earrings, and have great gloves on standby to hide ageing hands.

Hair

I love healthy, shiny, softly coloured hair that is neither too long nor too short, and soft bobs and hairstyles that move and bounce. I always recommend looking to Hollywood actresses for inspiration—Helen Mirren, Jane Fonda, Diane Keaton, Andie MacDowell and Jennifer Aniston. They always get it right.

- Never tease your hair, as it only makes your head, not your hair, look bigger.

- Shoulder-length or shorter styles will give you a more youthful appearance. If you're really keen to keep your hair long, use curls and waves to create movement.

- Colouring your hair black can be very harsh and ageing, regardless of your natural colour. Even natural blondes can look trashy if their hair is too yellow or overbleached. Choose light to mid-shades that look as natural as possible.

- Avoid tiger stripes and frizzy perms.

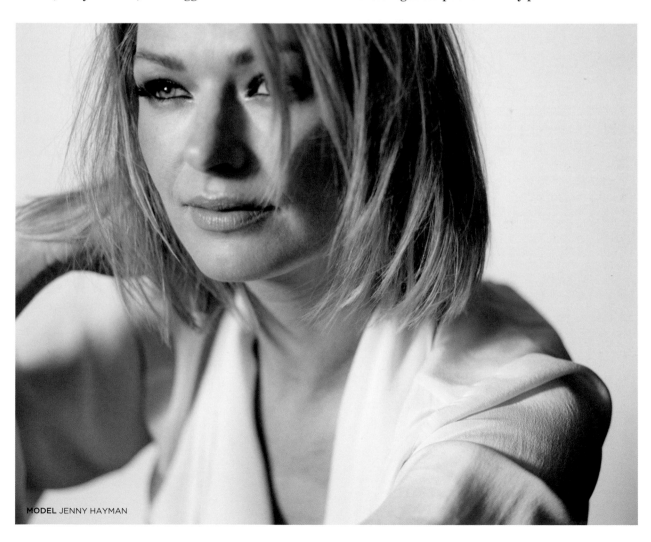

MODEL JENNY HAYMAN

Glasses

I'm going to talk about glasses frames, as this is the one accessory that affects both how you apply your makeup and what type you apply.

Glasses frames are not just about your eyesight—they can also be a great fashion accessory, and some women prefer them, in spite of all the advancements in vision technology, such as laser eye correction and contact lenses. I know models with perfect eyesight who wear frames as part of their look.

A frame can either highlight or disguise particular facial features around your eyes. This can work for or against you, depending on what you want to show or hide. Usually when we talk about glasses, we consider face and eye shape, but you can also use them as an accessory to bring colour into your face and to enhance and highlight your eyes.

If you wear prescription lenses in your frames, you should be aware of their effect. Depending on the prescription, they may either enlarge or reduce the appearance of your pupil size and the skin around your eyes. For example, if you're short-sighted, your lenses will make your eyes look smaller, while lenses for long-sighted people will have the opposite effect. Naturally this affects the look of your makeup. Glasses can amplify makeup mistakes, so make sure you get it right!

If you're still stuck in the '80s, and you're finding it hard to get over the fluorescent blue eye shadow that *may* have suited you back then, go for a more elegant eyeliner and use your glasses frames to get your colour fix instead.

FRAMES AND YOUR FACE

When choosing frames, first consider the shape of your face.

- **Small face**—small frames
- **Larger face**—large frames (it's that simple!)
- **Oval-shaped face**—suits most frames
- **Round face**—rectangular frames (round frames are a 'no-no' for obvious reasons)
- **Square face**—rounder frames

The next step is to figure out which frames will complement your other facial features.

- If you don't have great brows, choose glasses that cover them. If you *do* have great brows, choose glasses that allow them to be seen.
- Metal frames may be heavier to wear. Older women tend to look better in plastic frames.
- Do not wear round frames if you have hollow, sunken or round eyes.
- If you have baggy skin either above or under your eyes, pick a frame that can cut through the baggy area and obscure it (see the photo of Sarah in rectangular frames on page 81, bottom left).
- Look for glasses that don't sit too low on your face, which can make your face, and especially your eyes, look droopy. The bottom of the frames can also leave marks on your cheeks that take hours to disappear.
- Be careful of heavy frames and nose pads, which leave marks on your nose and, if you tend to sit your glasses on top of your head, get caught in your hair!

Unless you have an oval face, try to avoid wearing a frame the same shape as your face.

FRAMES AND YOUR MAKEUP

When buying glasses, use the eye colour charts as a guide (see page 44). These will give you the best match with your ideal makeup. Wear coloured frames that, when combined with your everyday makeup, will make your eye colour pop.

• Apply your makeup well, taking your glasses off and on to check every step.

• If you're scared of wearing colour on your eyes, go with an elegant and subtle makeup look and use the frames to add a splash of vibrant colour.

• The bolder and brighter your frames are, the more understated and elegant your makeup should be—try to stick to neutral tones.

• Some frames can cast a shadow around your naturally dark under-eye area, so be sure to conceal well. Before you continue with the rest of your makeup, try on your frames to make sure you've covered all areas.

• Curling your lashes well prevents them from touching the lenses and helps to make your eyes look more open.

• Keep your mascara clump-free—under the magnified lenses of your glasses, any clumps will be very noticeable.

• If you're using bold or graphic eyeliner on your lash line, you have to get it perfect, as your lenses may magnify your eyes. Make sure you blend your eyeliner well, otherwise it can appear very stark.

• Mineral foundation works beautifully around the nose area, where the nose pads sit—its light consistency means it won't wear off or mark as easily as oil-based foundation.

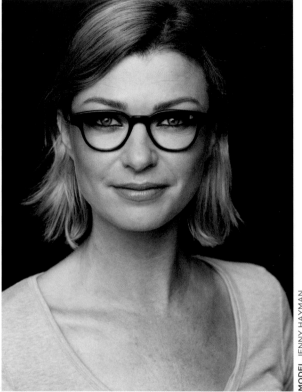

MODEL JENNY HAYMAN

• If you wear frameless glasses, go bolder and brighter with your makeup colours and make sure your brows make a statement.

• Don't rush into choosing frames. Pull your hair off your face and ask a friend to take photos with the flash off so you can check the effect of each style from all angles, especially side on.

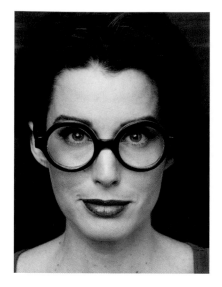

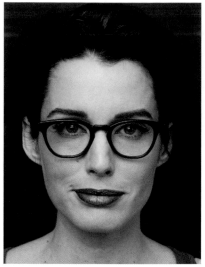

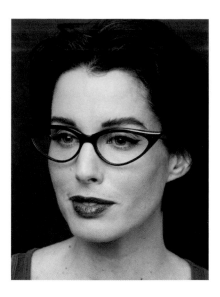

1 OWL

These create massive dints on the cheeks, so the only part of the face you see is the one that ages. If the lenses were magnified, these frames would be even more unflattering.

2 CLARK KENT

Although this style suits Julie, they will cause dints on her cheeks. They also draw the eye down to her cheeks, away from her eyes.

3 CAT'S EYE

The retro cat's eye shape is great if you want to show off a fantastic brow. Complement them with this great liquid eyeliner effect.

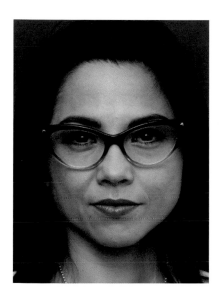

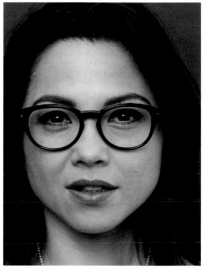

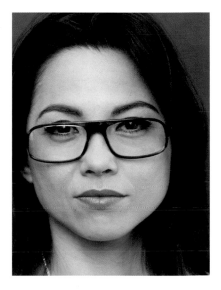

1 MODIFIED CAT'S EYE

The shape of this modified cat's eye is fine, but the dark frames cast a shadow over Rebecca's eyes, while the heavy black over her nose bridge does nothing for her.

2 CLARK KENT

This style suits Rebecca, and shows off her brows, as the frames sit a little off her nose. But they also sit a bit too low on her cheeks, and if the lenses were magnified, they'd be less flattering.

3 RECTANGULAR

These cut right through the eyes because of the way they're sitting on Rebecca's nose bridge.

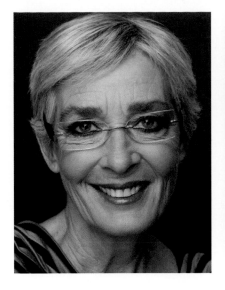 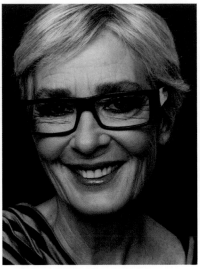 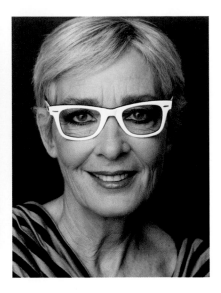

1 FRAMELESS

A perfect style if you're confident about your eye makeup and have beautiful brows to show off.

2 BLACK RECTANGULAR

This is a great shape, but it creates dark shadows. A different coloured frame would be more flattering.

3 MODIFIED CAT'S EYE

The heavy frame doesn't suit Robyn but the light colour really makes a difference to her face. Again, the frames sit heavily on the cheeks.

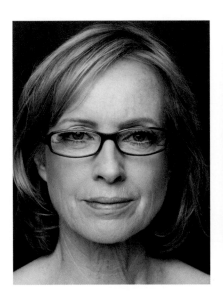 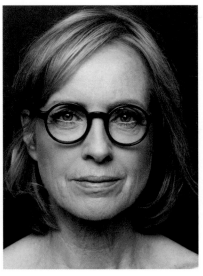 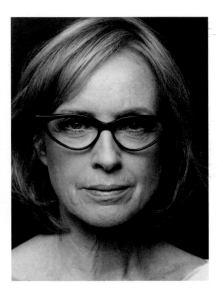

1 RECTANGULAR

This is my favourite shape for women concerned about the area under their eyes. It's a great style for Sarah, as it seems to lift her eyes and pull them apart. The width hides hollowing temples.

2 OWL

The owl shape enhances the under-eye area, giving Sarah hollow temples while covering her brows. These frames are also very heavy on the nose.

3 CAT'S EYE

This style creates a shadow too close to the eye and also covers up the brows and lashes, some of the most flattering parts of Sarah's eyes. A very fine gold frame would look fantastic on her.

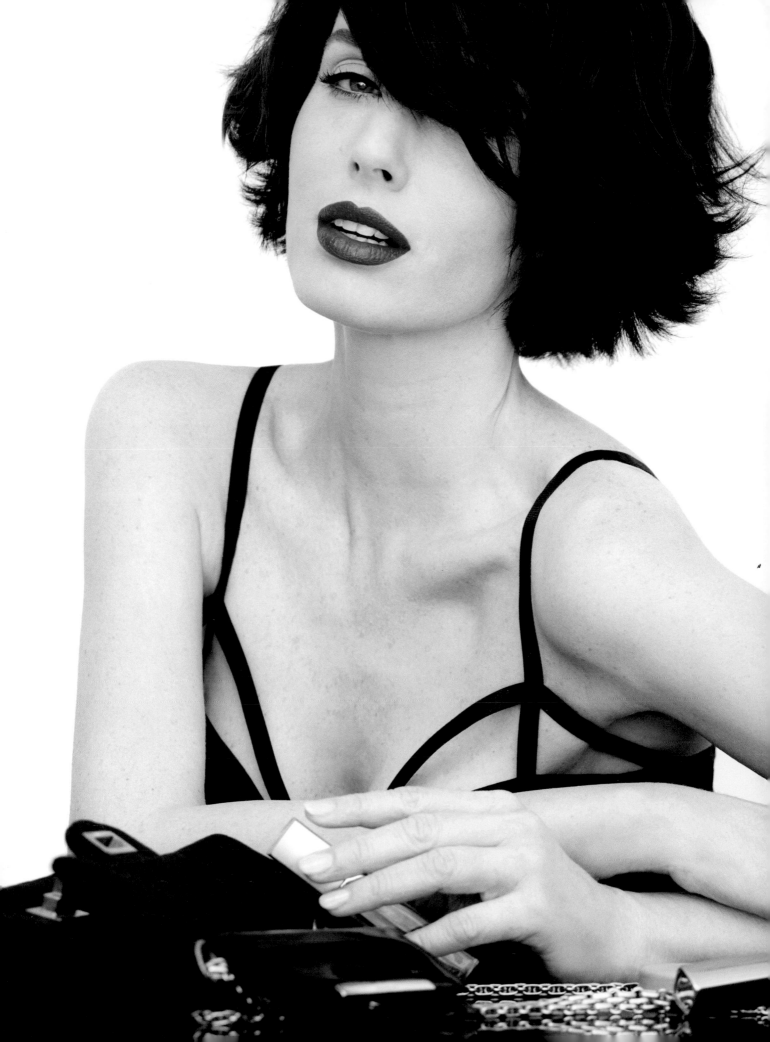

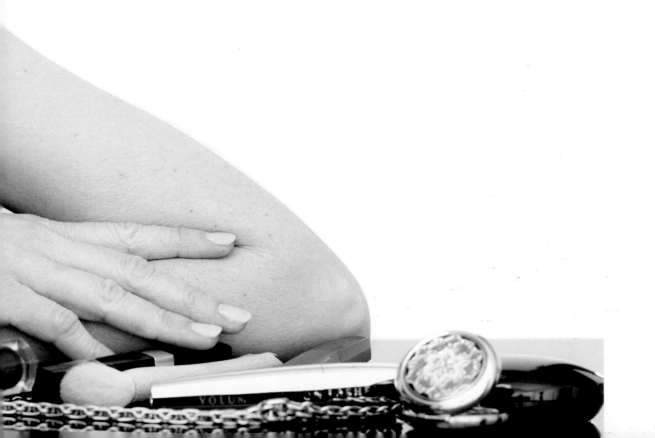

Looks

Scarlet Siren

EVEN THOUGH THIS LOOK IS STRONG, IT'S FABULOUS FOR DAY.

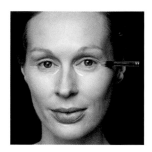

1 SKIN PREP AND FOUNDATION

Prep the skin with a water-based primer or moisturiser. Apply a sheer liquid foundation containing sunscreen all over, then concealer where necessary.

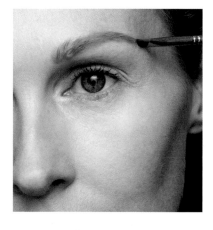

2 LASHES AND BROWS

Curl your lashes, and apply black mascara to your top lashes only. Define your brows.

If you don't have many lashes, or you find mascara a bit difficult to apply, have your eyelashes tinted.

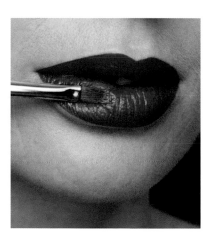

3 LIPS AND CHEEKS

Finish your foundation with a sheer translucent powder. Apply an intense orange-red lipstick, then a hint of blush if required.

Lip perfection like this requires constant maintenance.

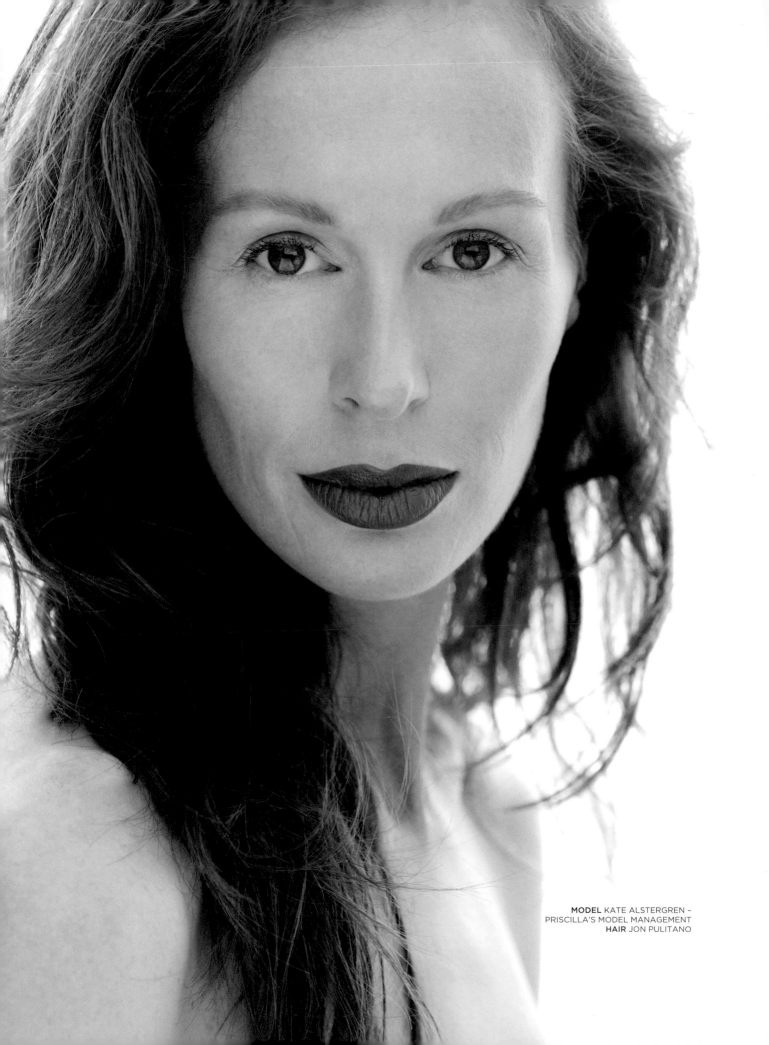

MODEL KATE ALSTERGREN –
PRISCILLA'S MODEL MANAGEMENT
HAIR JON PULITANO

Sheer Mahogany

A SOFT AND ELEGANT LOOK FOR EVENING.

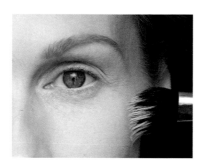

1 SKIN AND EYE PREP, AND BROWS

Prep the skin and eyes. Use a fibre-optic brush to apply liquid foundation, then define your brows. Apply a creamy white pencil to the inner rims of your eyes to open them up, and concealer where necessary.

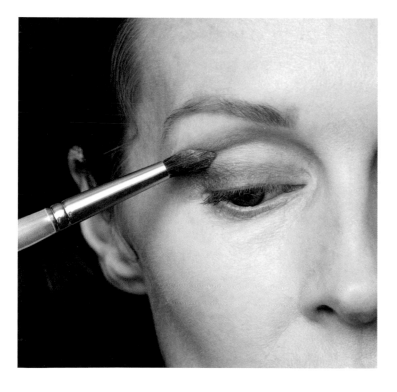

2 EYE SHADOW

With your eyelids well powdered, apply a warm brown eye shadow to the bottom half of the eyelid. As you age, your eyes become sunken, so don't extend the eye shadow into the socket, as dark shades will accentuate the depth. Instead, to lift and disguise the depth, apply a pale, skin-tone matte eye shadow directly into the eye socket.

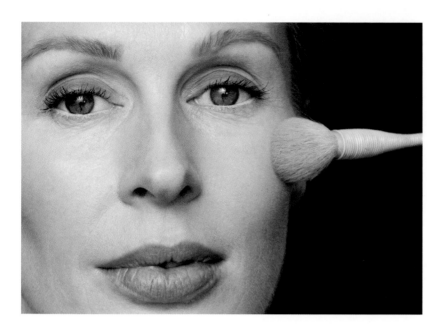

3 LASHES AND CHEEKS

Curl your lashes, and lift your eyes by applying lots of black mascara to the top lashes only. Use a kabuki brush to softly apply a peach-toned cream blush to your cheeks.

4 POWDER AND LIPS

Powder all over with a translucent powder to reduce shine and give the skin a beautiful velvety finish. Give your lips a healthy, youthful glow with a sheer mahogany lipstick. If you're wearing an open-neck top or dress, apply a touch of foundation to your décolletage to remove any redness.

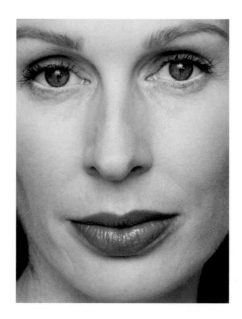

If you don't want to wear a lot of makeup and still look youthful and sophisticated, this is the look.

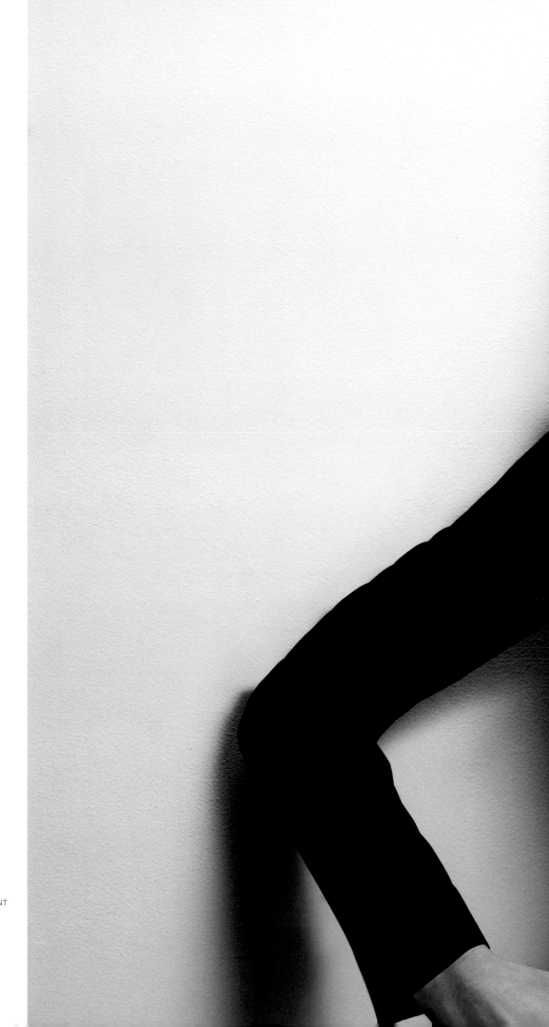

MODEL KATE ALSTERGREN –
PRISCILLA'S MODEL MANAGEMENT
HAIR JON PULITANO

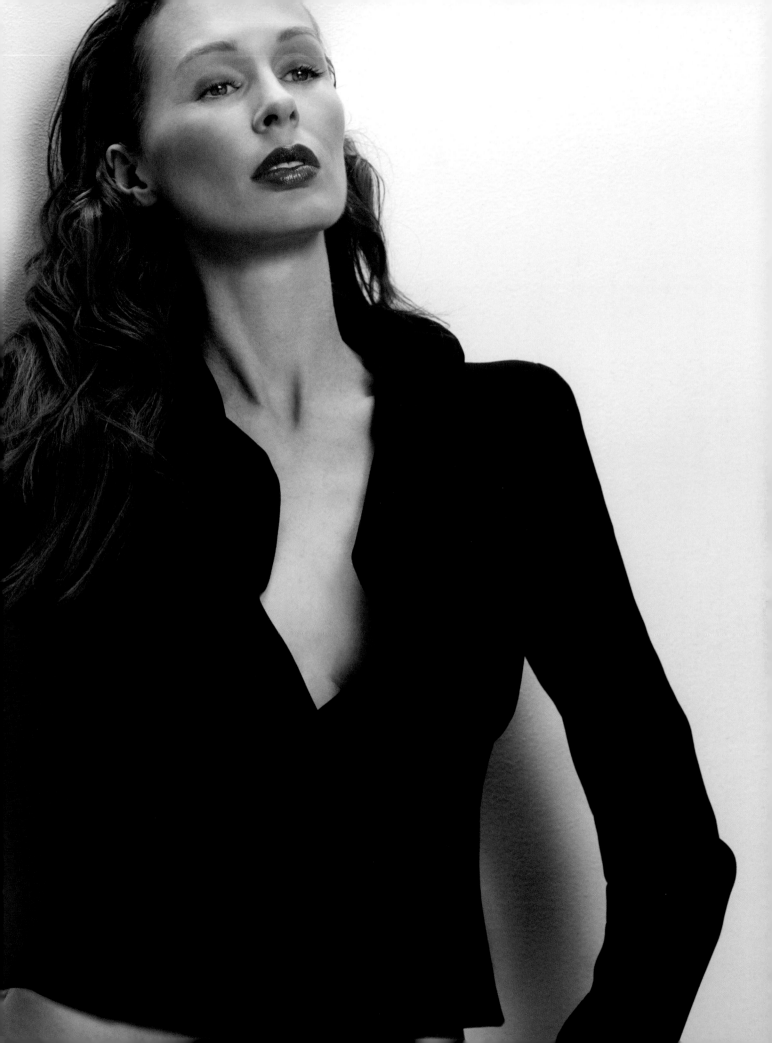

Luminous Intensity

A GREAT WAY TO SHOW OFF SUN-KISSED SKIN.

1 FOUNDATION, CONCEALER AND BLUSH

To give your face an extra glow, add a couple of drops of luminiser (see page 17) to your foundation and apply all over with a fibre-optic brush. Next, apply concealer where necessary, then a peach-toned cream blush to your cheeks. Blend well.

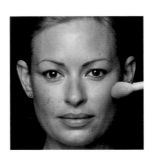

2 CONTOURING

If you want to have more defined cheeks, contour your cheeks and hairline (see pages 35–6). Remember, you can do this before or after you apply blush. Blend well.

3 EYE SHADOW

Make sure your eyelids are well powdered for optimum blending. Looking straight ahead into the mirror, create depth to your eyelids as shown by applying a warm brown matte eye shadow. To high-light the eyelids, apply a pale matte eye shadow. Shimmer will only accentuate fine lines.

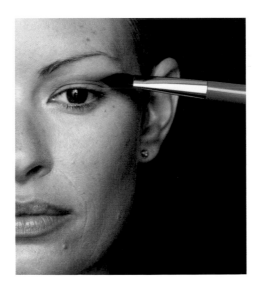

Start with a lighter shade of eye shadow then build up to a darker one. This will cut your blending time in half.

4 BROWS AND LASHES

Define and fill in your brows, curl your lashes and apply lots of black mascara to your top and bottom lashes. To enlarge your eyes, apply a pale flesh-coloured pencil onto the inner rim of each eye.

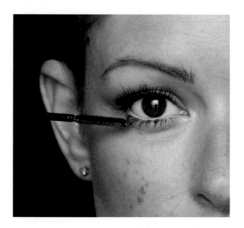

I have lightened shayna's brows temporarily with a brow mascara. If you have any stray grey eyebrows, this is a great way to disguise them.

5 FALSE EYELASHES

If you feel confident, cut a full false lash in half and apply it to the outer edges of your natural lashes (see page 64). The lash glue may appear white at first but don't worry, it dries clear. Notice the lash applicator I'm using—once you've tried this miracle tool, you'll never apply lashes the normal way again.

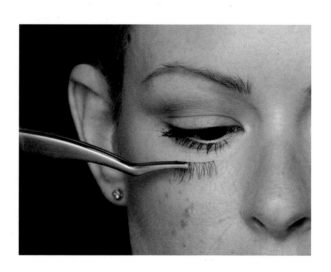

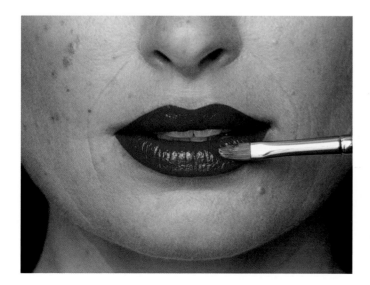

6 LIPS

Use a lip brush to apply an orange-red lipstick. Blot off any excess.

MODEL SHAYNA ROBERTS –
PRISCILLA'S MODEL MANAGEMENT
HAIR JON PULITANO

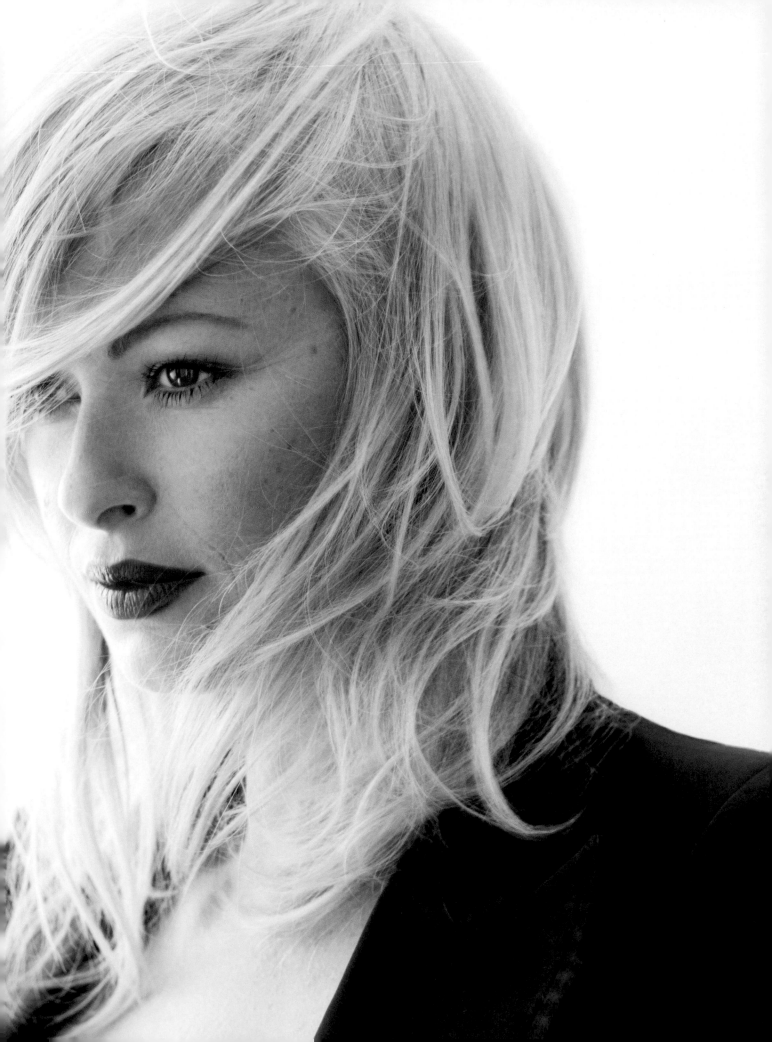

Sultry Blonde

AN UNDERSTATED SMOKY EYE, FOR ANY OCCASION.

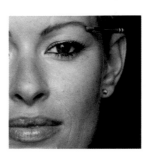

1 FOUNDATION, BROWS AND LASHES

Use a foundation brush to apply liquid foundation. Define the brows, curl the lashes and line the inner rims of the eyes with a dark chocolate kohl pencil that's not waterproof.

I quickly tinted shayna's eyelashes— a great trick if you struggle to put on mascara.

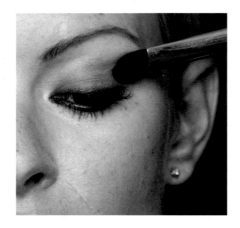

2 EYELINER AND EYE SHADOW

Line the entire lash line with the same kohl pencil and smudge with an eye shadow brush. Then blend the edges with a softer brown matte eye shadow into the eye socket and under your bottom lash line. For a beautiful winged effect, blend out the edges.

3 POWDER, BRONZER AND LIPS

Powder all over with a sheer translucent powder. Softly apply a matte bronzer to your cheeks and hairline. Finish with a nude lipstick.

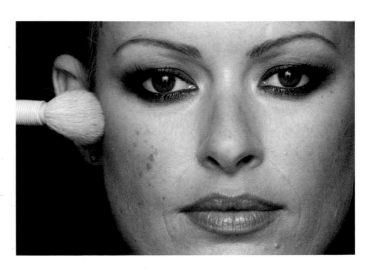

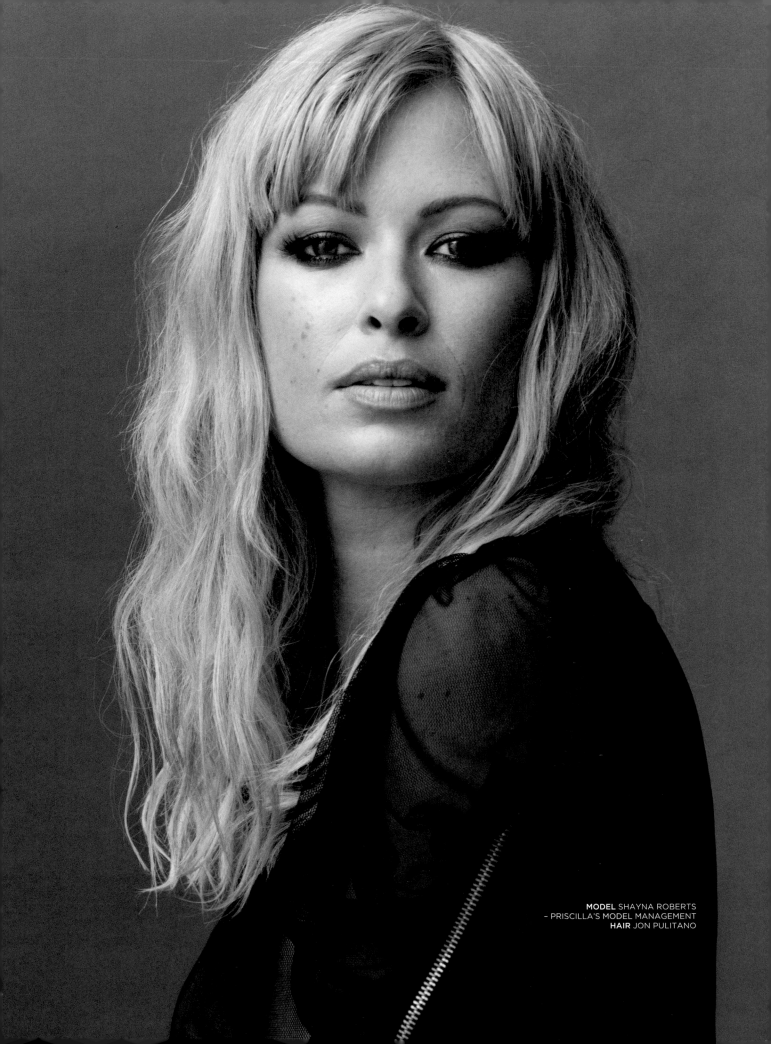

MODEL SHAYNA ROBERTS
– PRISCILLA'S MODEL MANAGEMENT
HAIR JON PULITANO

Green Ice

JENNY HAS FABULOUS SKIN WITH JUST A HINT OF PIGMENTATION.

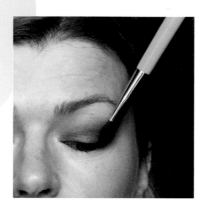

1 PREP AND EYE SHADOW

Prep your eyelids, and make sure they're well powdered for optimum blending. Apply a golden bronze eye shadow to the eyelid, blending to just slightly above the brow bone. Notice I'm holding the brush vertically—most of the eye shadow is on the tip of the brush, so holding the brush this way ensures that the colour intensity will be on the lash line, fading towards the top of the lid.

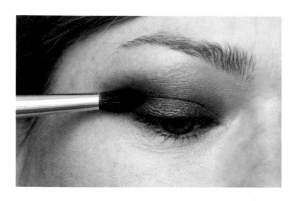

2 EYE SHADOW

Use a smaller brush to apply a deep mahogany eye shadow in the same way as in step 1, but this time don't blend up as high. Then, holding the brush horizontal, blend out to the side from the outer corner of the eye.

3 FOUNDATION, BROWS AND EYELINER

Clean up any fallout from under the eye, and apply foundation all over. Define the eyebrows, and apply concealer where necessary. Apply a chocolate brown eye pencil to the inner rims of each eye.

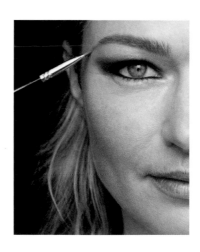

Lowering the eyebrow reduces the fullness of the eyelid. Here I've used an eyebrow brush with a shadow matched to Jenny's brow colour. This has a subtle but noticeable effect.

4 EYE SHADOW

Take the golden bronze eye shadow you first applied to the top eyelid. While looking up, blend softly along the lower lash line. Then highlight the inner corner of the eye with an intense gold pigment.

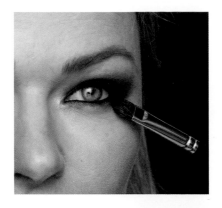

It's important to use only a matte shade of eye shadow under the eye, as any form of sheen or shimmer will accentuate any fine lines.

5 EYES AND CHEEKBONES

Smudge the same chocolate brown kohl pencil along the top lash line, keeping it thicker and more intense on the outer edges. Blend well. Curl your lashes, and apply lots of black mascara to your top lashes only. Lightly contour the temples and under the cheekbones, as shown (see also page 35).

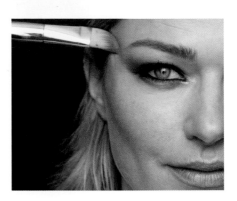

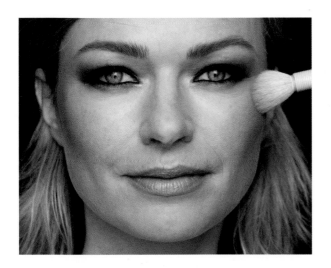

6 POWDER, BLUSH AND LIPSTICK

Apply a light translucent powder all over, and then a soft pink powdered blush to the cheeks. Notice how high I'm applying the blush. Finish off with a sheer pink lipstick.

When applying eye shadow for this look, follow these three steps.
1 Use a bigger brush to apply the lightest colour to the eyelid, and into the socket.
2 Use a slightly smaller brush to apply the mid-colour from the eyelash line to the top of the eyelid.
3 Use a smaller brush again to apply the darkest colour, and to help smudge the colour into the eyelash line.

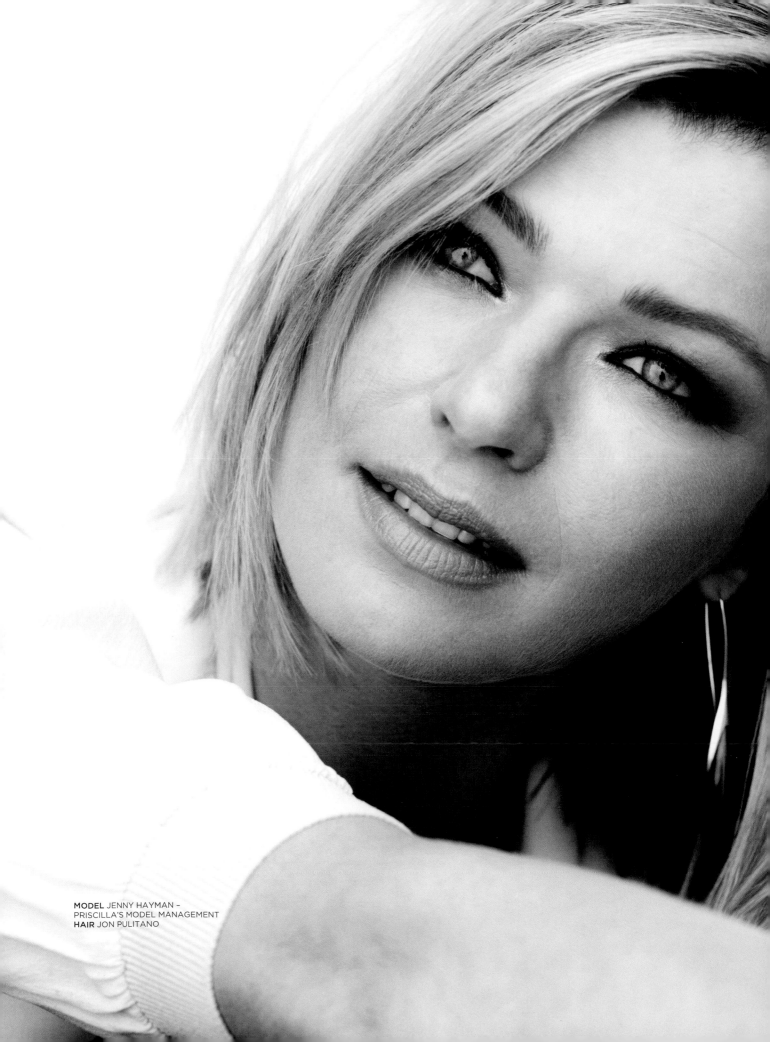

MODEL JENNY HAYMAN –
PRISCILLA'S MODEL MANAGEMENT
HAIR JON PULITANO

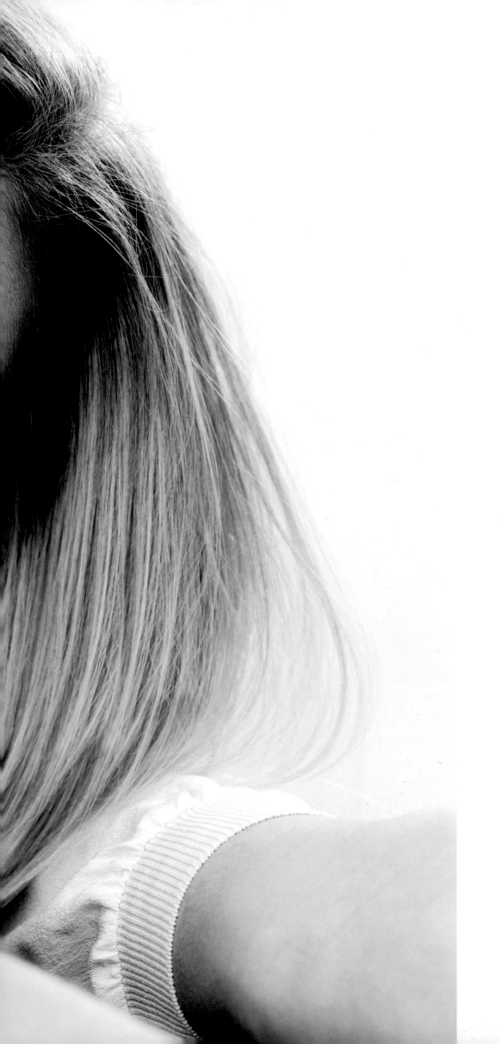

Belle de Jour

I WANT TO ACCENTUATE JULIE'S ALMOND-SHAPED EYES.

1 SKIN PREP, POWDER AND EYELINER

Apply a liquid foundation all over, and concealer where necessary. Powder all over with a translucent powder, but pay particular attention to the eyelids—this will prevent the eyeliner from smearing. Make sure you apply foundation to your eyelids to knock out any blue-red tones. Apply sticky tape as shown, then use a black gel eyeliner to apply a very fine line across your top eyelid. Flick it up onto the sticky tape, then gently peel off the tape.

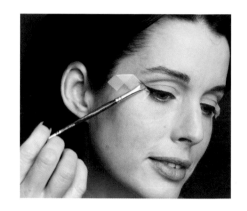

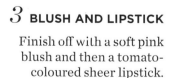

2 LASHES AND BROWS

Curl your eyelashes, apply lots of black mascara to the top lashes, and define your brows.

3 BLUSH AND LIPSTICK

Finish off with a soft pink blush and then a tomato-coloured sheer lipstick.

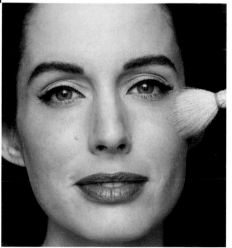

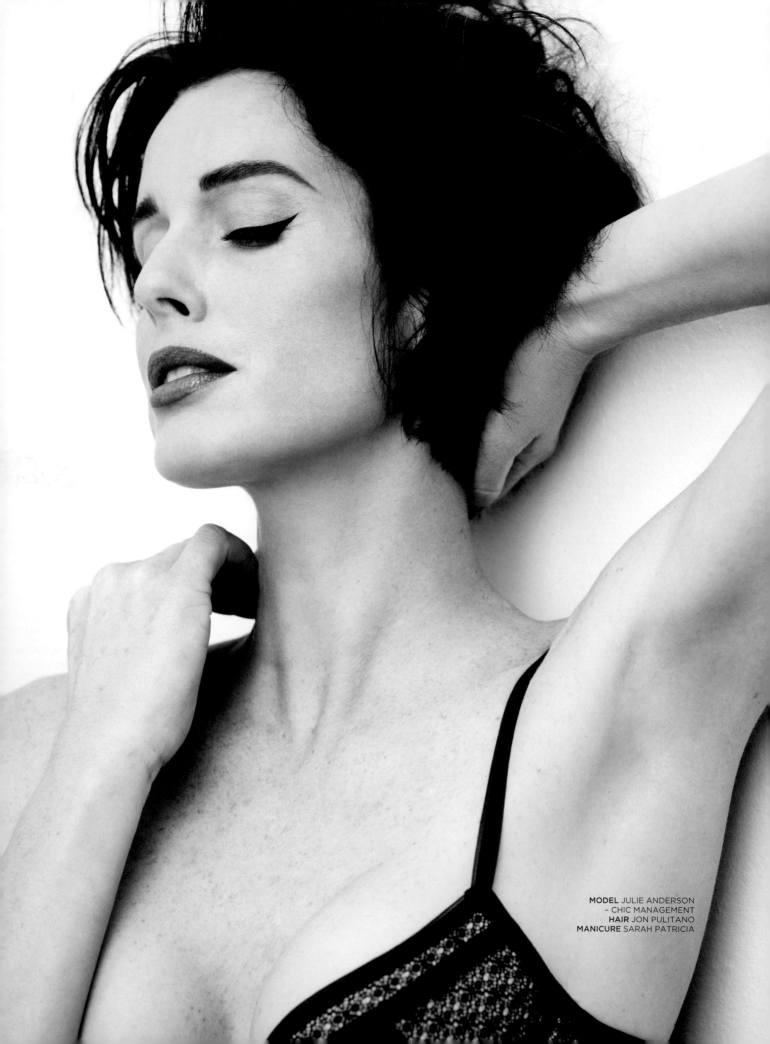

MODEL JULIE ANDERSON
– CHIC MANAGEMENT
HAIR JON PULITANO
MANICURE SARAH PATRICIA

Honeysuckle Rose

SHADES OF VIOLET INTENSIFY JENNY'S GREEN EYES.

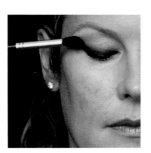

1 EYE PREP AND EYELINER

I'm going for a strong eye, so I'm doing the eyes first. Prep your skin, apply foundation to the eyelid only and lightly powder it for optimal blending. Heavily apply a dark violet kohl pencil, about half a centimetre wide, along the top lash line. Then use an eye shadow brush to blend the pencil outwards.

2 EYE SHADOW

Use a violet matte eye shadow to wash over the whole lid to just under the brow bone, keeping the intensity at the outer corner.

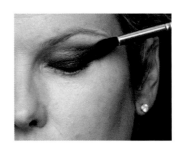

3 EYELINER

Use a black kohl pencil to create a triangular shape in the outer edge of the eye. Holding a small oval-tipped brush vertically, blend outwards.

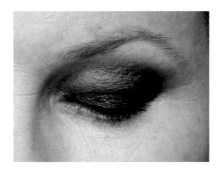

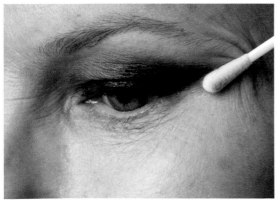

4 FALLOUT

With a little cleanser or foundation on a cotton bud, remove any fallout from the corner of the eye. (To create the illusion of fantastic bone structure, remove everything from under the imaginary line that runs from the corner of the nose to the corner of the eye.)

5 FOUNDATION, CONCEALER AND BROWS

Apply liquid foundation all over, and concealer where required. Pencil in your brows where necessary. Jenny has naturally over-arched eyebrows that give the illusion of puffy eyelids. Lowering the arch and extending the brow gives her eye more lift—I have only done one brow so you can see the difference. We need to darken the brow bone, not highlight it. Use a creamy white pencil to line the inner eye—a great way to open up and refresh the eyes and remove redness.

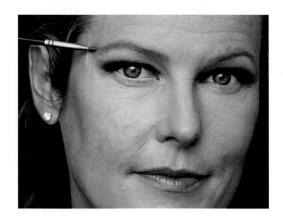

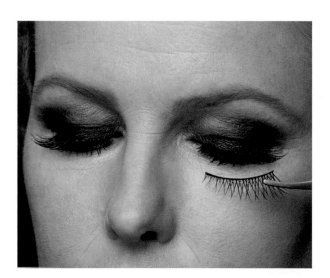

6 EYES AND POWDER

Lightly smudge grey matte eye shadow along the lower lash line, apply lots of black mascara top and bottom and, if you're feeling confident, apply a 3/4 false lash with an eyelash applicator. Powder your T-zone.

7 CONTOURING AND BLUSH

Contour the hairline, and apply blush to the cheeks. Jenny has a natural contour under her cheekbone, so I'm applying only a subtle contour to the temples. A luminous cream blush keeps her skin fresh and beautiful. Watermelon lipstick completes the look.

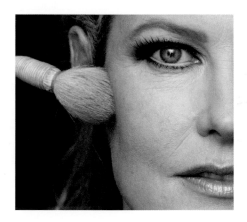

As Jenny has minimal lines on her face, I can afford to use a luminous blush.

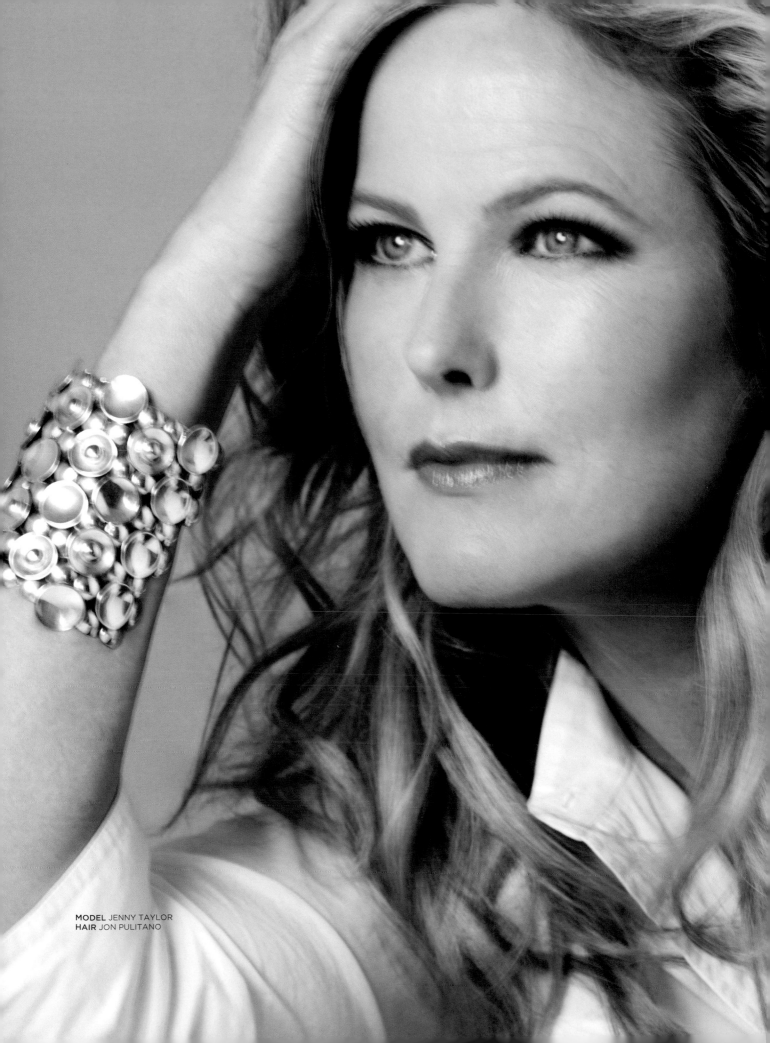

MODEL JENNY TAYLOR
HAIR JON PULITANO

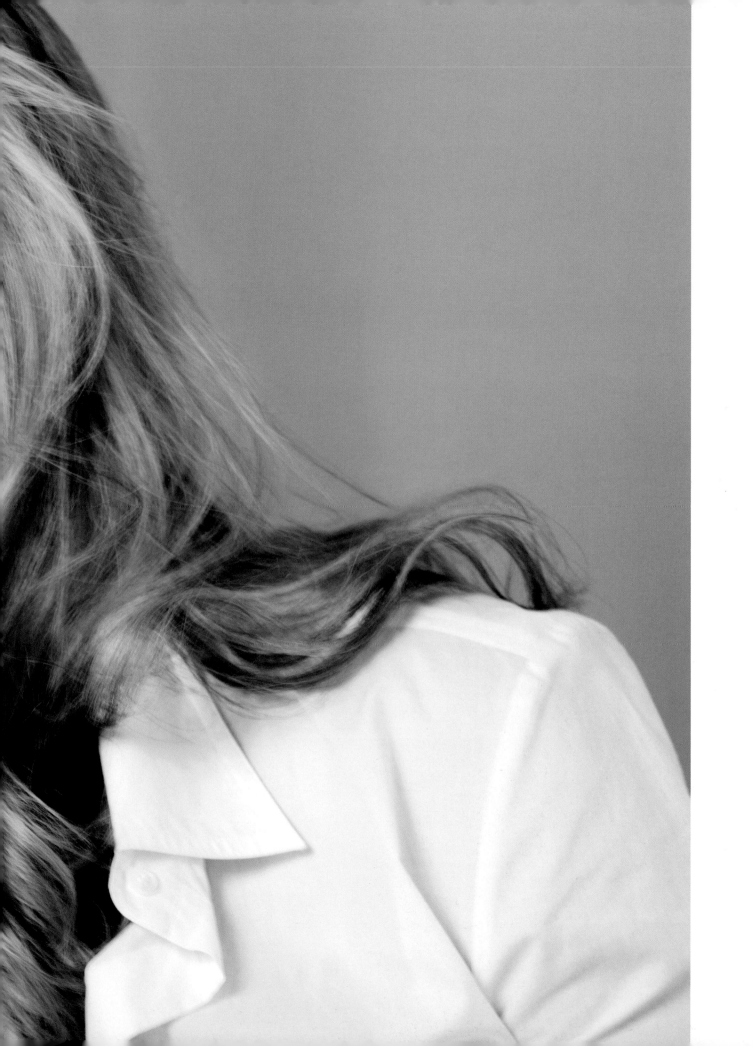

Rock Chic

WHO SAYS THIS LOOK IS FOR THE UNDER 18S?

1 SKIN PREP AND BROWS

Prep your skin and pluck any stray brows. Robyn has dream eyebrows—they're full and not over-arched. Apply a liquid foundation all over the face, and concealer where necessary. I'm not using any powder, as I want to keep Robyn's skin luminous.

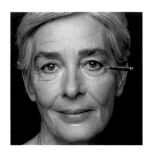

To conceal any grey eyebrow hairs, use a coloured brow mascara (see page 18).

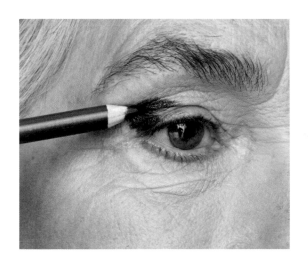

2 EYE PREP AND EYELINER

Powder your eyelids only. Looking straight ahead into the mirror, apply a chocolate brown kohl pencil to the area of the eye you'd like to recede. Remember, dark colours recede or 'push back', while light colours come forward.

3 BLENDING

Looking down, use an eye shadow brush to blend the pencil into a soft C-shape, then intensify the lower lash line with more chocolate brown kohl pencil.

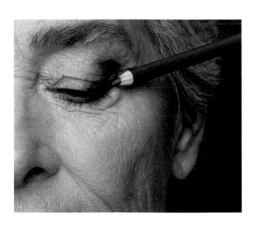

Don't start applying any eye shadow until you've fully blended this eye pencil.

4 EYE CONTOURING

To help lift the under-eye area, apply the same kohl pencil to the inner corner and inner rim. Then use a small angled brush to smudge the pencil into the lash bed. Use a dark brown matte eye shadow to blend the lower lash line.

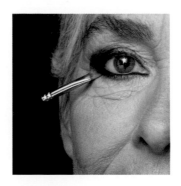

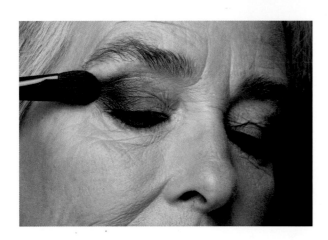

5 EYE SHADOW

While looking down, brush a light brown wash over the whole eyelid, then use a darker brown matte eye shadow to intensify the outer corner of the eye. Blend well.

6 LASHES, MASCARA AND BLUSH

Curl the lashes and apply black mascara to your top and bottom lashes (I used a mascara wand to comb the lashes and remove any clumps), and apply a rose blush.

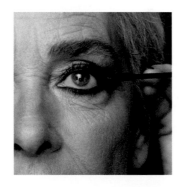

If your lashes are sparse, get some lash extensions (see page 62), or try using latex to apply a few single lashes yourself.

With a strong eye like this you can look hot for day or evening – even just wearing the right accessories with a simple white shirt or a denim jacket.

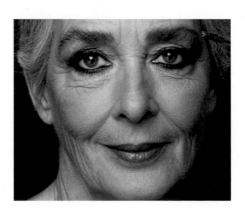

7 BROWS AND LIPS

Finish off with a light brown brow mascara and mahogany lipstick.

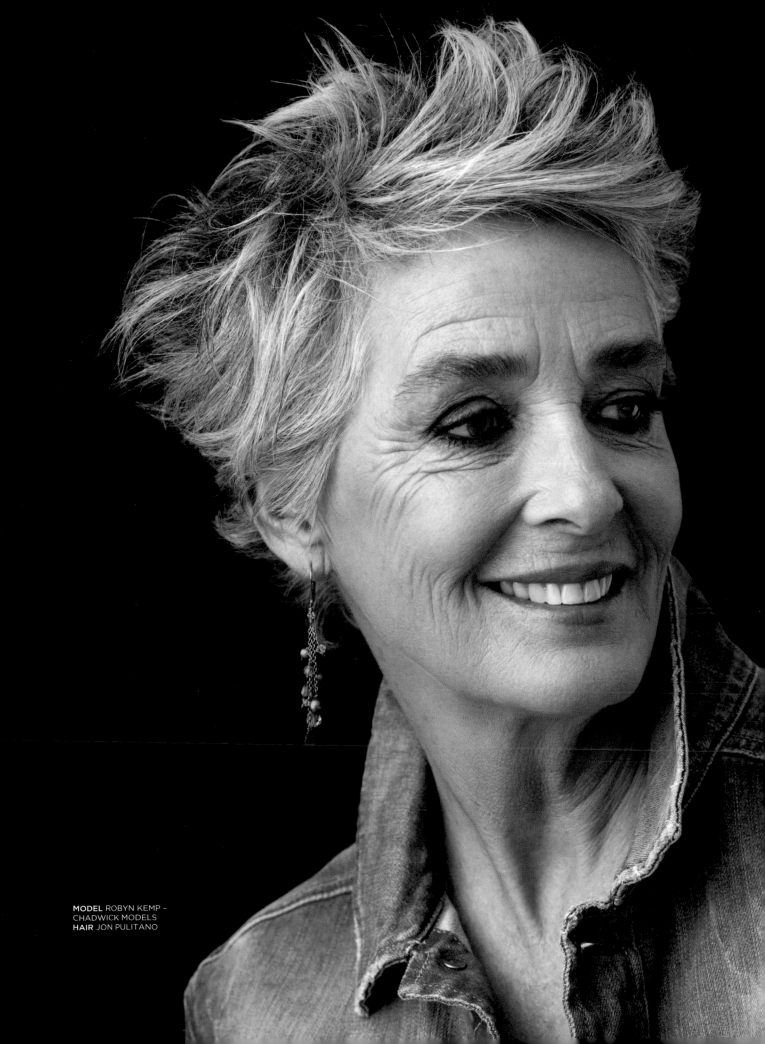

MODEL ROBYN KEMP –
CHADWICK MODELS
HAIR JON PULITANO

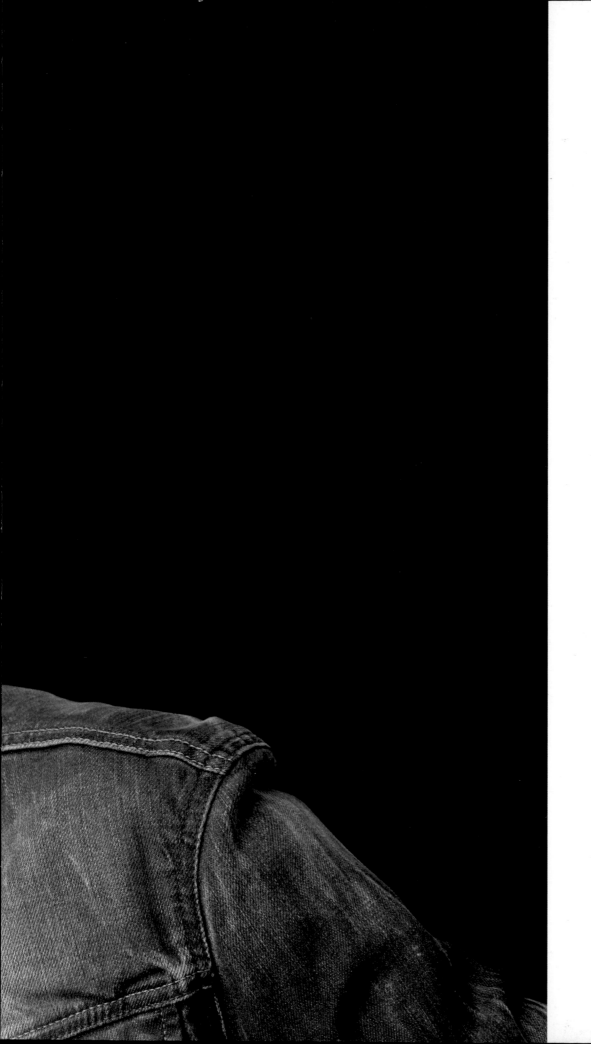

Tea Rose

A FEMININE LOOK THAT'S PRETTY AND ELEGANT.

1 PREP AND FOUNDATION

Apply lip balm to your lips so that, by the time you do your lips, they're already nice and soft. Apply a creamy liquid foundation all over, and concealer where necessary, then lightly powder the eyelids. To help conceal any redness, apply a creamy white pencil to the inner rim of the eye.

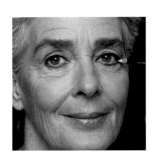

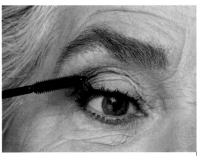

2 EYE SHADOW

Apply matte eye shadow in a cream shade over the whole lid to just under the brow bone. Apply a grey matte eye shadow only to the edge—lightly extend it out towards the temple and gently up to the brow bone.

3 LASHES AND MASCARA

Curl the lashes and apply black mascara. Fill in the brows where necessary.

4 CHEEKS AND LIPS

Apply a soft rose blush and a sheer nude lipstick with a lip gloss. For a slightly more dramatic look, add a few extra individual lashes to the outer corners.

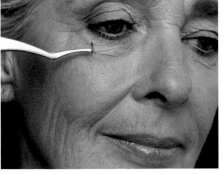

When you have a lighter lip, you can afford to make your cheeks and eyes stronger.

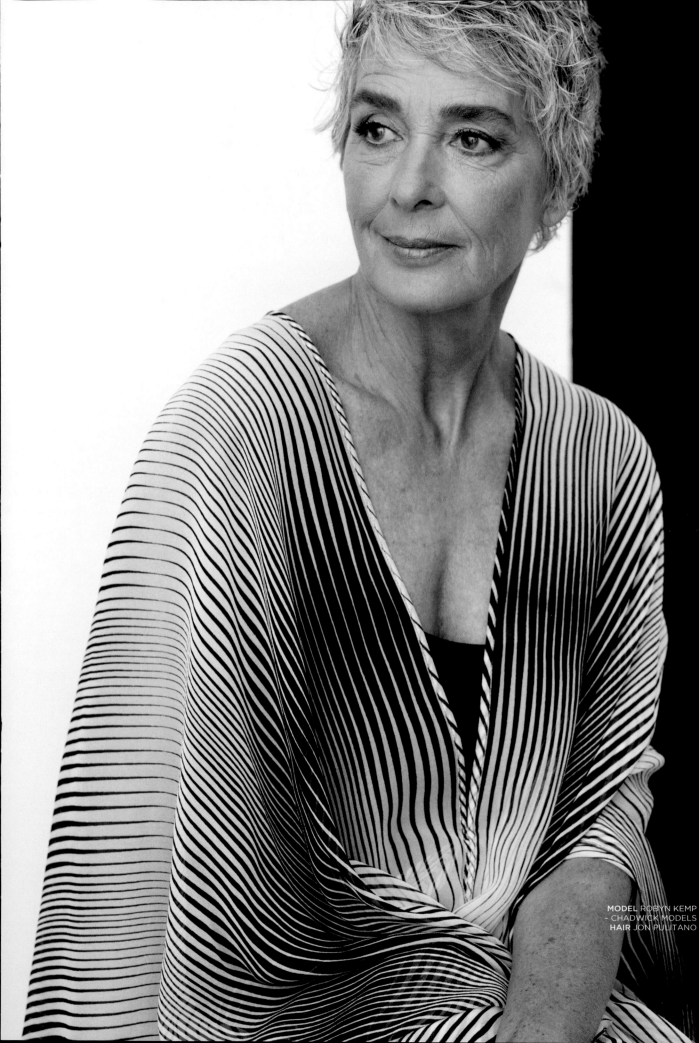

MODEL ROBYN KEMP
- CHADWICK MODELS
HAIR JON PULITANO

French Marigold

TRY THIS LOOK WHEN YOU NEED A LIFT.

1 SKIN PREP AND EYELIDS

Prep the skin. Apply liquid foundation all over, and concealer where necessary. Powder the eyelids, then apply a grey matte eye shadow just underneath the brow bone. Use a shadow in a paler cream shade to lift and brighten the inner socket.

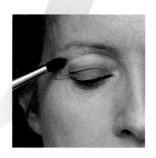

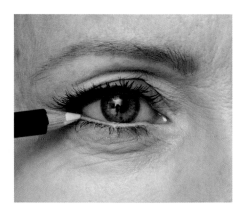

2 EYELIDS, BROWS AND LASHES

Smudge some grey matte eyeliner pencil a third of the way in from the outer corners of the eye. Lining just the outer third will lengthen the eye, but if you line all the way across, your eyes will look too round. Smudge the eyeliner and define the brows. Curl the lashes, and apply lots of black mascara. Powder the T-zone.

3 LASHES

Apply a creamy white pencil to the inner rims. If you're confident, apply some false lashes. Finish with black mascara on the bottom lashes.

If your eyes tend to be a bit droopy, avoid the creamy white pencil on the inner rims, as it can drag down your eyes.

4 CONTOURING

Use a contouring brush to contour the cheeks and hairline (see pages 35–6). Blend well.

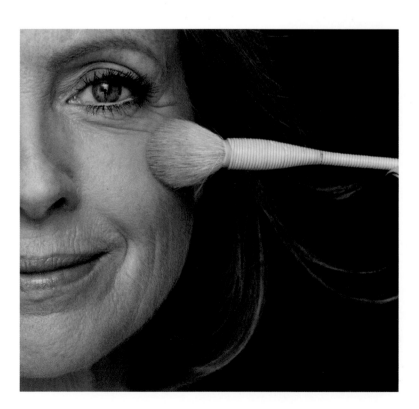

5 CHEEKS AND LIPS

Finish off with a rose cream blush blended onto the top of your cheeks with a kabuki brush, then apply a peach nude lipstick.

This look is a trick I pull out when someone's jetlagged or sleep-deprived.

MODEL SARAH GRANT –
CHADWICK MODELS
HAIR JON PULITANO
MANICURE SARAH PATRICIA

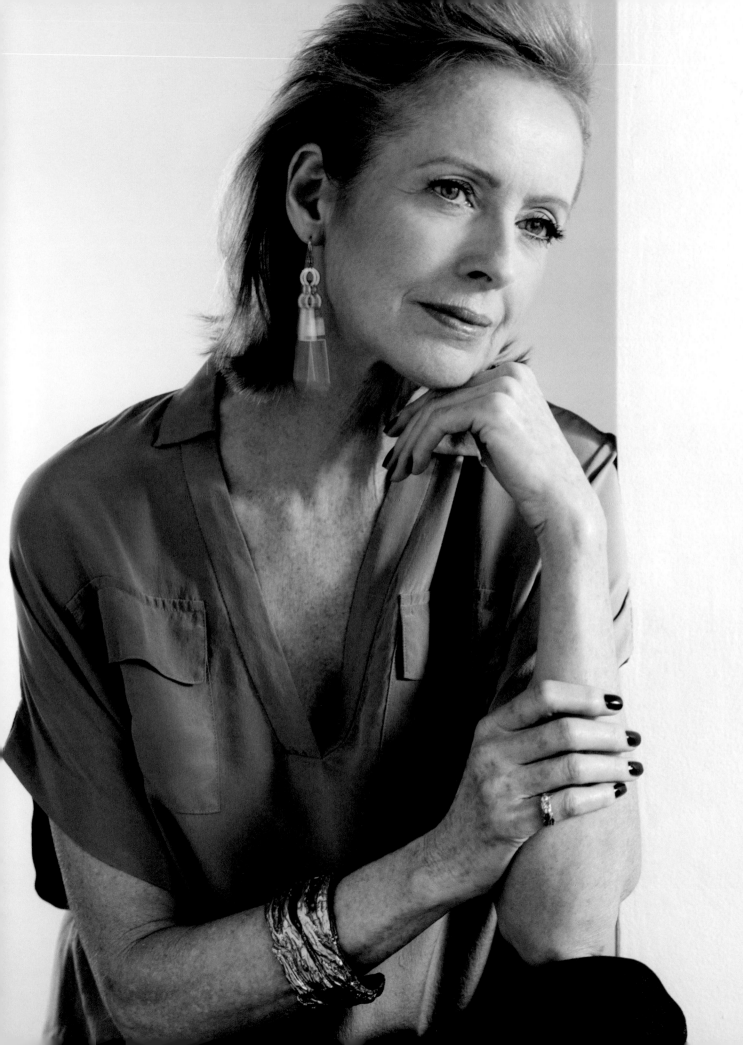

Creamy Peach

COVER UP LINES UNDER THE EYES WITH THIS DRAMATIC LOOK FOR NIGHT.

1 SKIN PREP, BROWS AND EYE SHADOW

Prep your skin. Use a liquid foundation all over, and concealer where necessary. Powder all over and define the brows. Apply light brown matte eye shadow across the lid and just below the socket line (make this your base colour eye shadow). Apply dark brown matte eye shadow on the outer edges. This will help 'lift' your eyes.

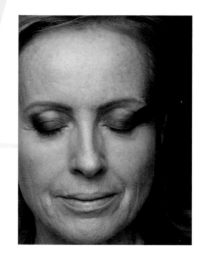

Be careful not to take the dark brown colour into the inner part of the eye socket, as it will make your eyes look too sunken.

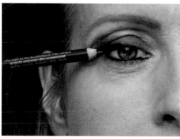

2 EYELINER

Use a black kohl pencil to line the inner rim of the eye and the outer edge of the top eye line.

3 EYE SHADOW

Use a black eye shadow and a fine brush to smudge a fine line on both the lower and upper lash lines. Work close to the lash line to help set the pencil and prevent it from running. It also gives a soft edge. Remember to lightly extend the eye line across the whole lash line, but keep it extremely fine.

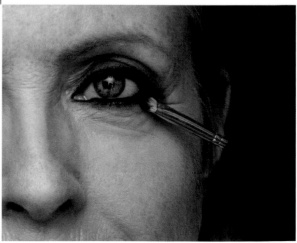

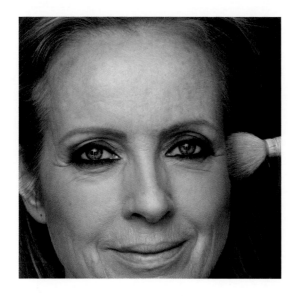

4 CONTOURING AND BLUSH

Apply a soft peach powder blush, then contour the cheeks and the hairline (see pages 35–6)—a must for a high or large forehead.

5 LASHES

Curl the lashes, and add black mascara to the top and bottom lashes. Finally, apply individual lashes to the top, but only if you think you need them.

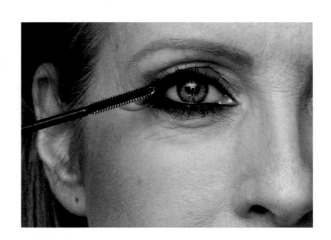

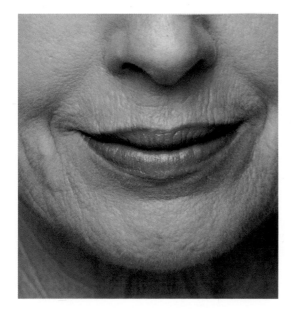

6 LIPS

Finish off with a soft mahogany lipstick that is very close to your natural lip colour. Mahogany is perfect, as it gives the illusion of whiter teeth.

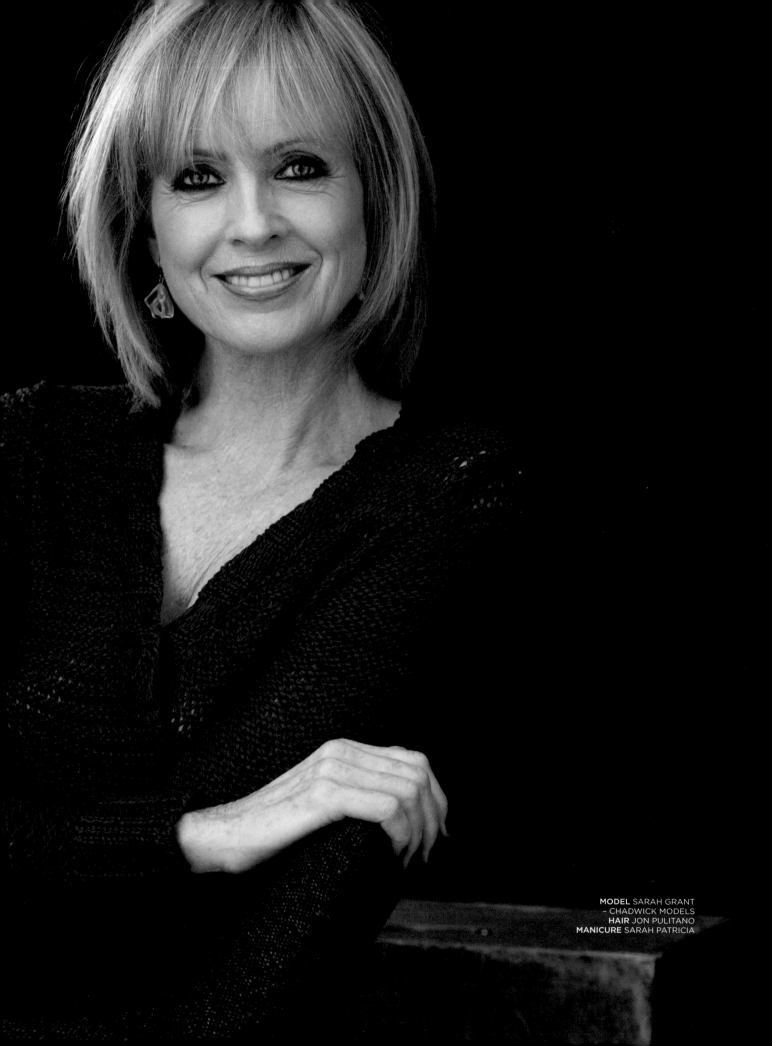

MODEL SARAH GRANT
– CHADWICK MODELS
HAIR JON PULITANO
MANICURE SARAH PATRICIA

Tawny Tigress

WEAR EYELINER AND LINGERIE AND LOOK HOT.

1 FOUNDATION, CONTOURING AND HIGHLIGHTING

To give your skin a beautiful glow, apply a liquid foundation with a few drops of gold metallic luminiser. Apply concealer where necessary, then contour the cheekbones and hairline.

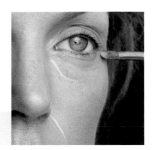

Wet your brush to stop the shimmer from falling on your skin, as it will enhance any lines.

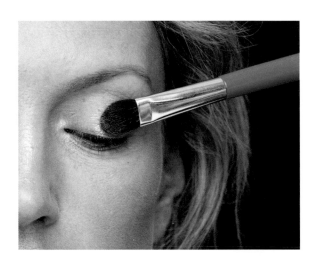

2 EYELINER, LASHES AND BROWS

Use a gold shimmer to highlight the inner corner of the eye, the centre of the eyelid, the cupid's bow, down the centre of the nose and lightly on the top of the cheekbone. Then take a black gel eyeliner and smudge the finest line along the top eyelash bed. If you don't feel confident, use a black eye shadow and smudge it. To lift the eyes, curl the lashes and apply lots of black mascara to the top lashes. Apply a few single false lashes to the outer corner.

3 CHEEKS AND LIPS

Apply a creamy white pencil to the inner rims of your eyes and define your brows. Finish with a light peach cream blush and sheer light pink gloss.

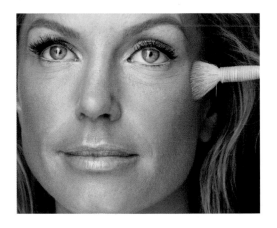

If your skin tends to be too shiny during the day, first blot the oil with blotting papers, then apply a translucent powder.

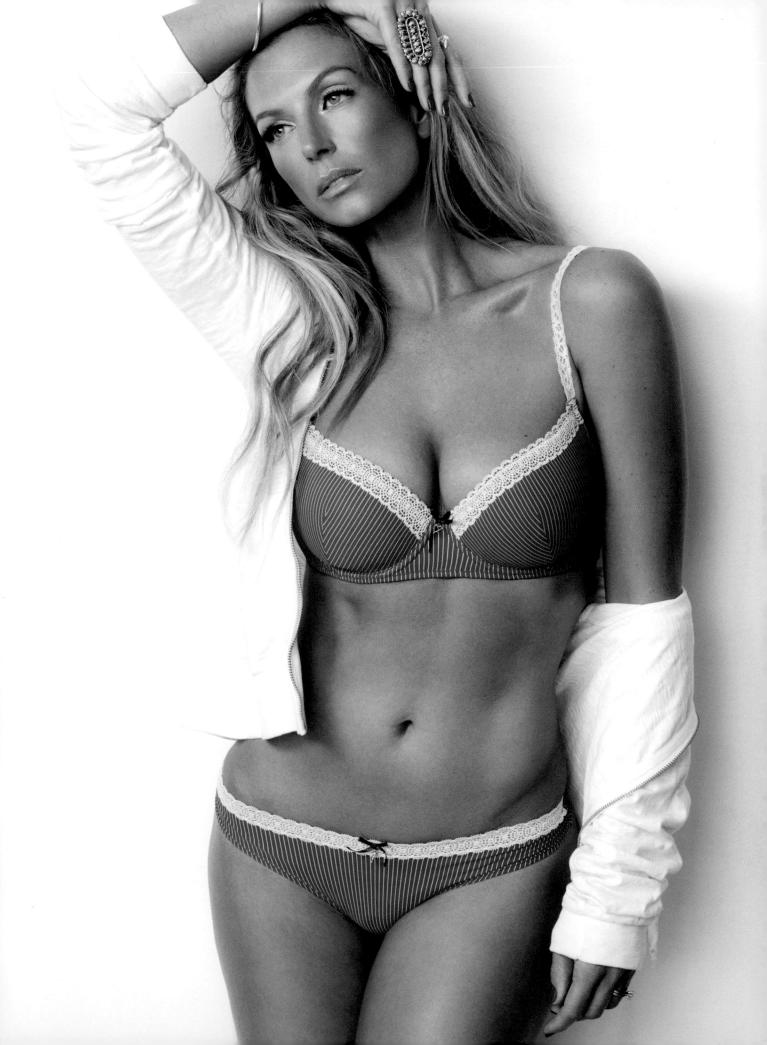

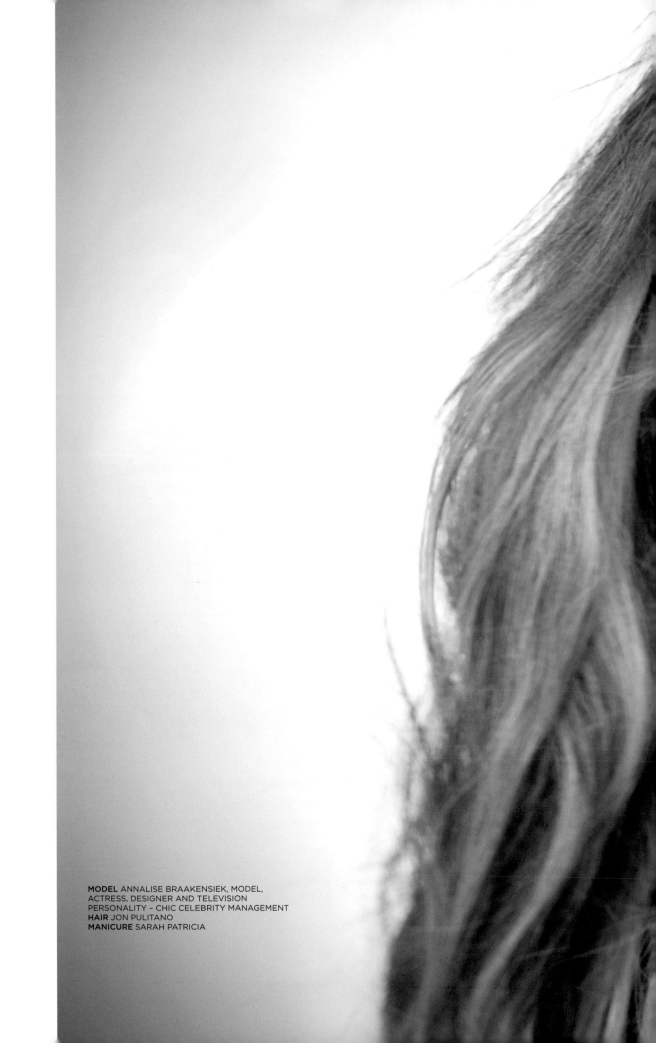

MODEL ANNALISE BRAAKENSIEK, MODEL,
ACTRESS, DESIGNER AND TELEVISION
PERSONALITY – CHIC CELEBRITY MANAGEMENT
HAIR JON PULITANO
MANICURE SARAH PATRICIA

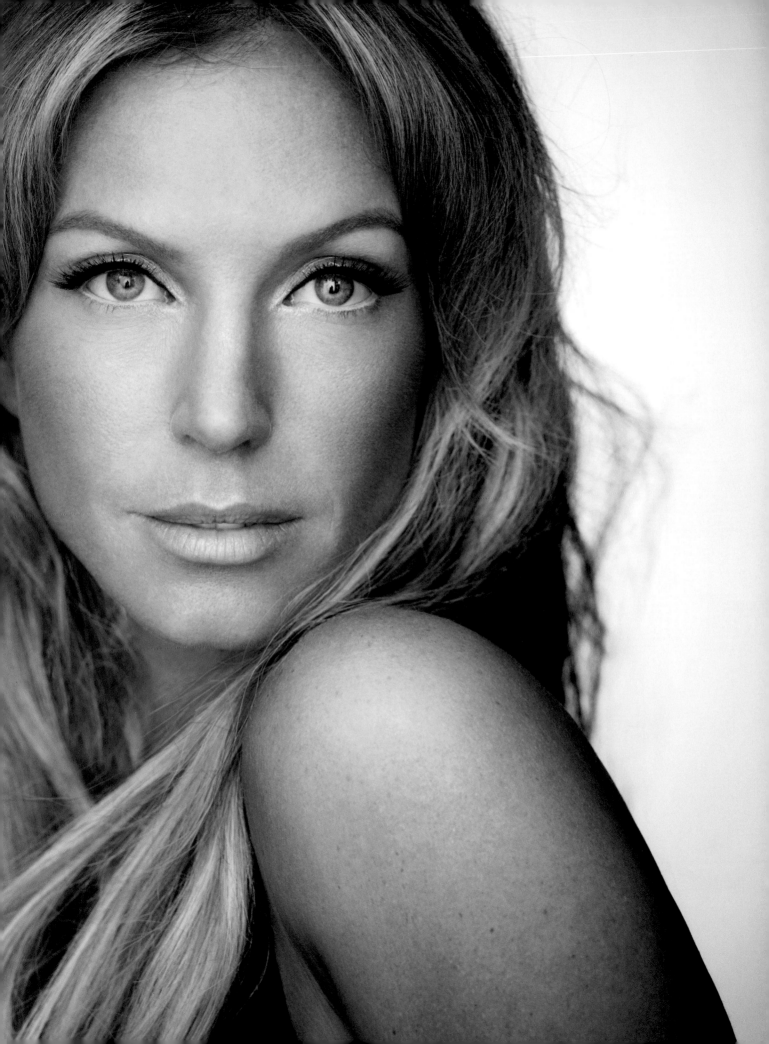

White Magnolia

I MOVED THE SPOTLIGHT FROM MARY'S SLIGHTLY RED CHEEKS TO HER LIPS.

1 SKIN PREP, FOUNDATION AND POWDER

Apply creamy foundation all over, blending down to the neck. Let it soak into the skin for a few minutes. This will cover the majority of the redness, so you'll need less concealer. Conceal where necessary and define the brows. Lightly powder all over.

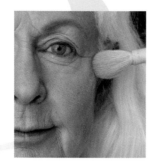

If you have any blemishes or redness, do not use concealer first, as the foundation brush will take it off anyway—excessive use of concealer is never the answer for a perfect base.

2 EYE SHADOW

Apply grey matte eye shadow over the entire lid, to just above the socket line. Looking straight ahead into the mirror, darken the fold of skin you wish to push back and lift—remember, dark eye shadow pushes the skin back while light will enlarge it (see page 42).

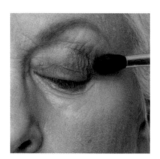

Don't apply matte grey on the inner corner of the eye area, as it will make the eye look even darker and more deep-set—not flattering!

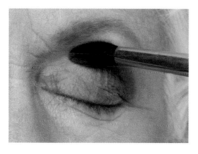

3 EYE SHADOW

Apply cream-coloured matte eye shadow to the darker socket of the inner eye. This is the area where you must avoid all dark shadows.

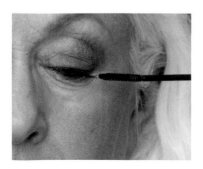

4 CHEEKS AND LASHES

When you have naturally pink cheeks, it's important to knock out the red. In Mary's case, her natural pink is in the wrong area. Once I removed the red, I applied a soft rose blush to her upper cheeks to give her a lift and make her look more youthful. Curl the lashes, then apply black mascara to the top lashes only. If you're confident, apply single false lashes. Alternatively, get lash extensions, or have your eyelashes tinted.

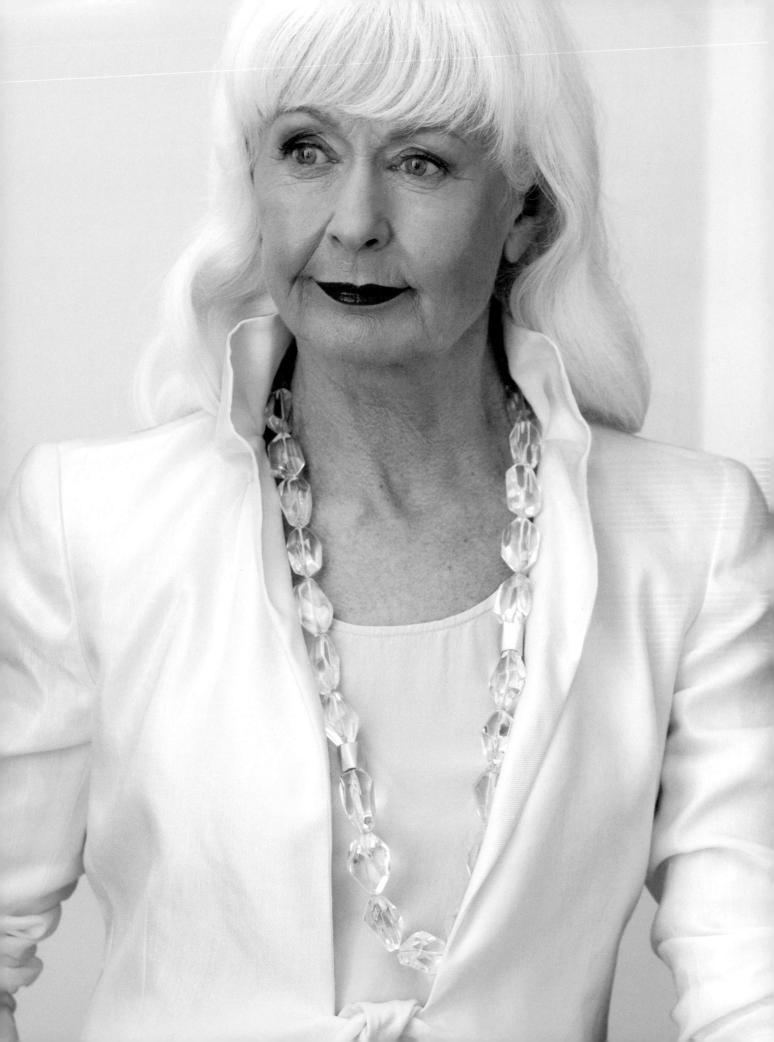

MODEL MARY SHACKMAN, ARTIST
HAIR JON PULITANO

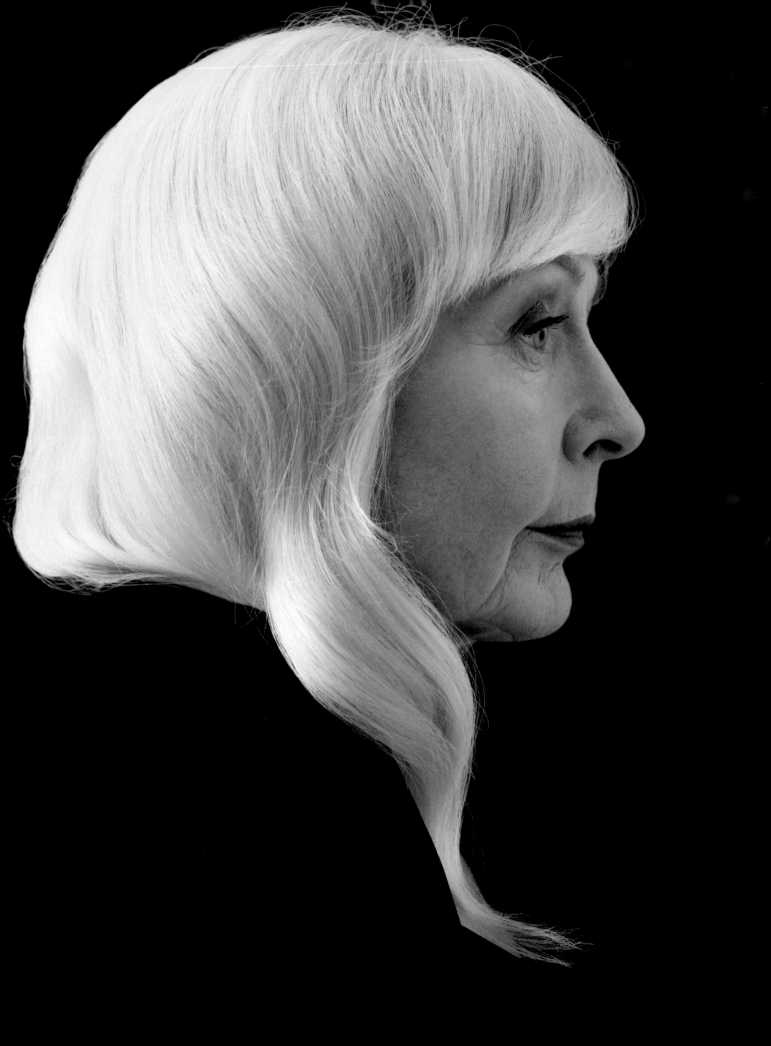

Serene Queen

A SOFT BUT GROOMED AND ELEGANT LOOK.

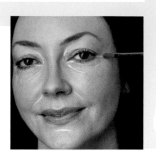

1 SKIN AND EYE PREP, AND BROWS

Prep your skin (see page 24). Leona has amazing skin, so she needs only a tinted sunscreen and a hint of concealer. Apply a light wash of foundation to the eyelids, then lightly powder this area only. Define the brows—I've lowered the arch of Leona's brows, as an over-arched brow can make the eyelid look puffy.

2 EYELINER AND LASHES

Apply creamy white eyeliner to the inner rims of the eyes, curl the lashes and apply lots of black mascara to the top and bottom lashes.

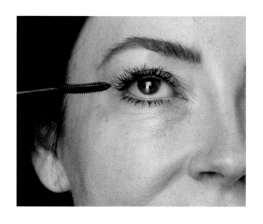

3 EYELINER, CHEEKS AND LIPS

Use a hooked eyeliner brush to smudge black gel eyeliner really close to the lash line. On the outer corner, slightly flick out the line. To finish, use a shell-pink cream blush and matching lip shade. This is one of my favourite 'Timeless' looks.

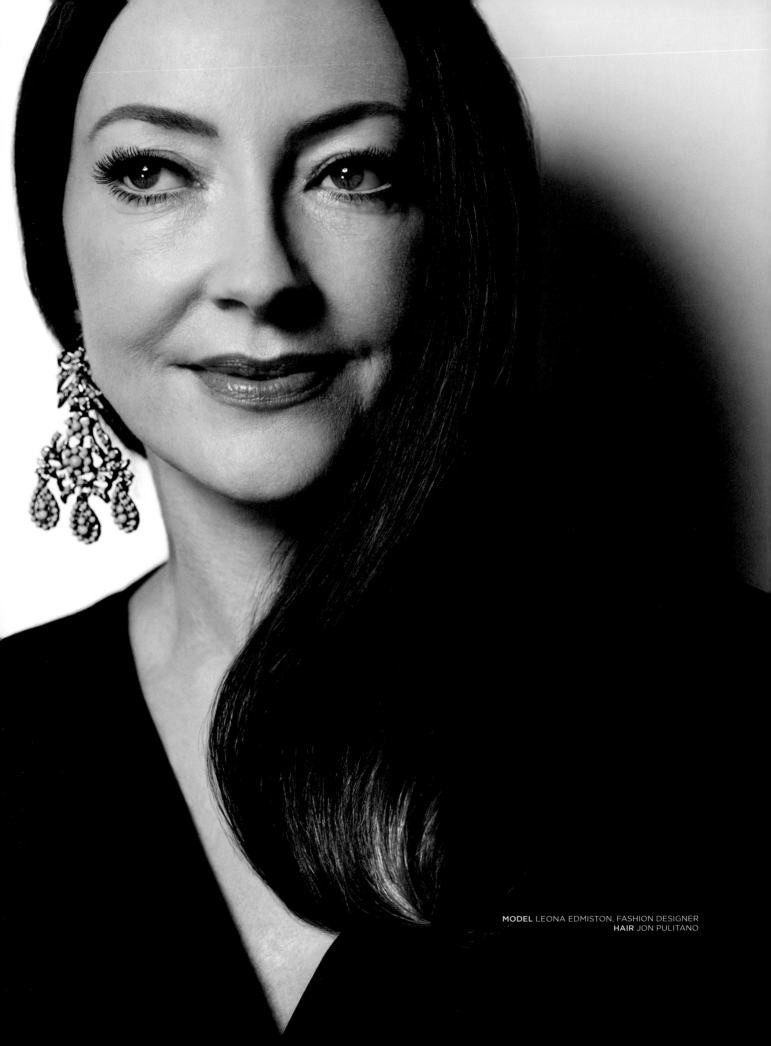

MODEL LEONA EDMISTON, FASHION DESIGNER
HAIR JON PULITANO

Velvet Shimmer

A NATURAL LOOK FOR WOMEN WHO DON'T WANT TO WEAR MAKEUP.

1 SKIN PREP

Prep the skin, and apply a pale but warm liquid base foundation all over, then concealer where required.

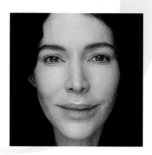

If, like me, you have pigmentation on your neck, apply foundation to conceal it.

2 BROWS, EYE PREP AND HIGHLIGHTING

Define and clean up your brows, then comb them up and fill in where necessary. Powder the eyelids. Apply creamy white pencil to the inner rim of the eye. Highlight the cupid's bow and inner corner of the eye with a pale gold shimmer powder.

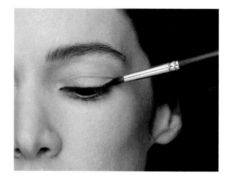

As I'm quite long in the face, contouring would make me look skeletal, so I've avoided it.

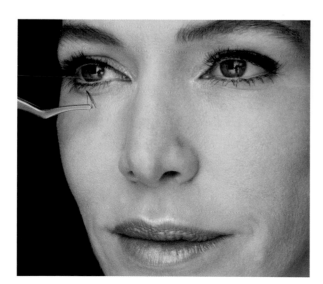

3 EYELINER, LASHES AND LIPS

Using a black gel liner, smudge the finest line along the top lash bed. Apply a shimmery cream-based pink blush to your cheeks. Curl your lashes. Apply black mascara top and bottom, and apply single lashes to fill in any gaps. Finish off with lip gloss.

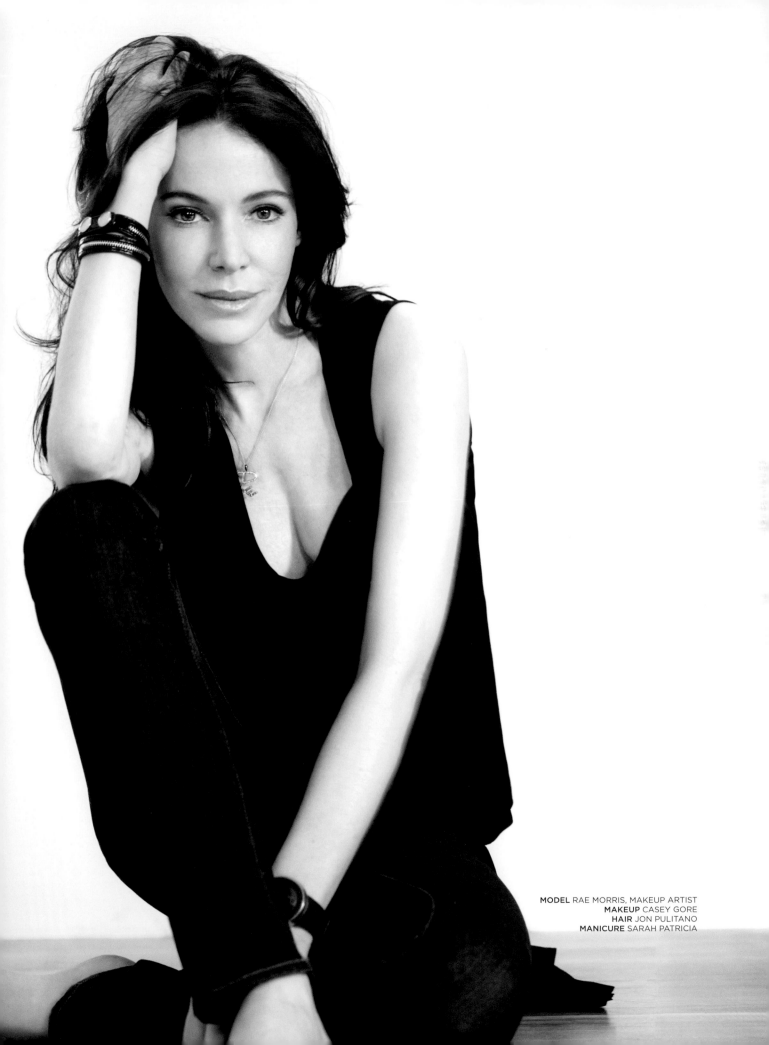

MODEL RAE MORRIS, MAKEUP ARTIST
MAKEUP CASEY GORE
HAIR JON PULITANO
MANICURE SARAH PATRICIA

Matinée Idol

I WANTED TO LIFT OLGA'S EYES AND MAKE THEM LOOK MORE CAT-LIKE.

1 SKIN PREP AND BROWS

Prep your skin. To help cover any skin blemishes, buff a thick, creamy foundation into the skin, all over, with my Deluxe Buffer brush. Apply concealer where necessary, then clean and define your brows. Lightly powder the T-zone.

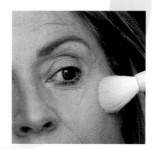

If your foundation starts to crease around your eyes, just use your fingertip to smooth it back out.

2 EYE SHADOW AND EYELINER

Apply a dark navy blue eye shadow in a triangular shape across the eyelid towards the outer corner of each eye. Make it thicker as you get to the outer corner of the eye. Draw a fine line across the eyelash bed with navy blue gel eyeliner and thicken it towards the outer corner of the eye. Do a little flick at the end if you like.

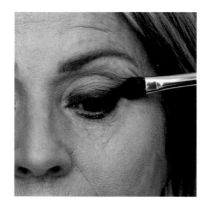

You can use pencil eyeliner instead, but I prefer gel, as it's waterproof. To help blend any eye shadow, use a clean brush loaded with translucent powder.

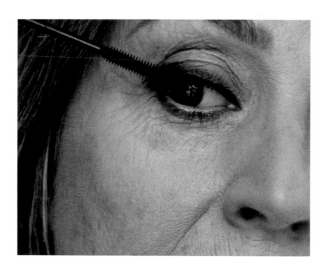

3 LASHES

Use a creamy white eyeliner on the inner rim of the eye. Curl your lashes and apply black mascara to the top lashes.

4 BOTTOM LASH LINE

Using the same navy blue eye shadow, elongate the eye by lining the bottom lash line from the lowest point of the eye to the outer corner of the lash. Gently smudge the shadow along the outer third of the eye. If you feel confident, apply single lashes.

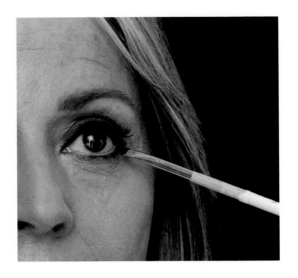

5 CONTOURING AND BLUSH

Contour your cheeks (see page 35). Shade the hairline and cheekbones, then apply an apricot blush.

6 HIGHLIGHTING AND LIPSTICK

Highlight the cupid's bow and the inner corners of your eyes with a gold shimmer. Finish with a dusty rose lipstick.

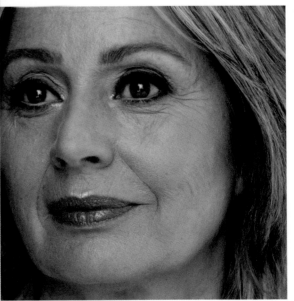

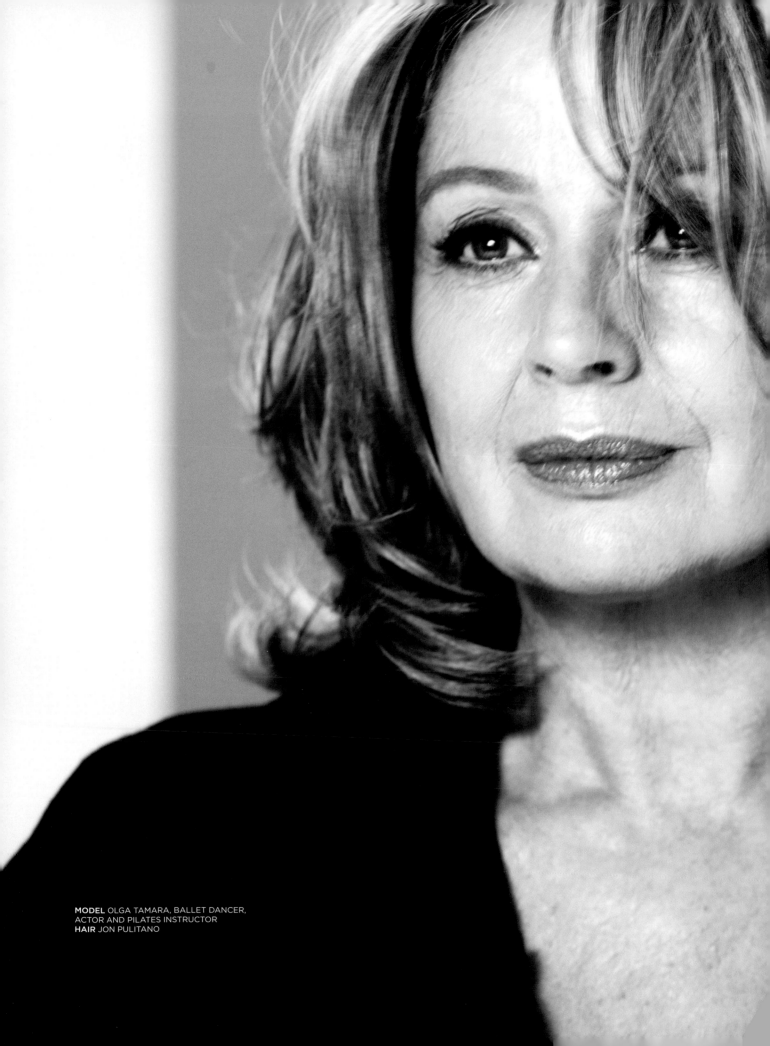

MODEL OLGA TAMARA, BALLET DANCER, ACTOR AND PILATES INSTRUCTOR
HAIR JON PULITANO

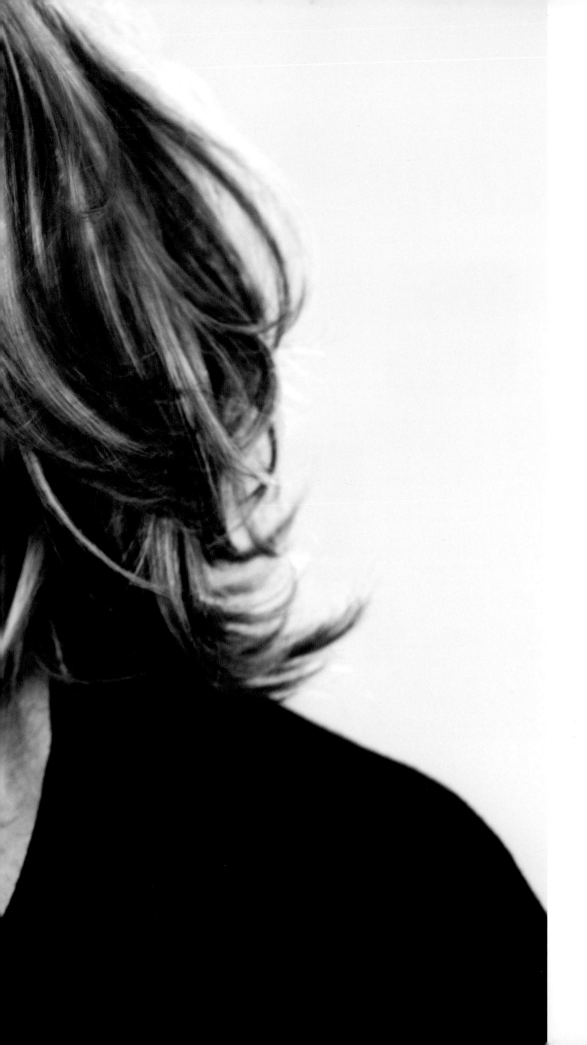

Mata Hari

THIS LOOK IS FANTASTIC FOR HIDING FINE LINES ON THE EYELID.

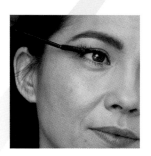

1 SKIN PREP, BROWS AND LASHES

Prep the skin. Apply foundation all over, and concealer where necessary. Clean and define your brows and curl your lashes. Apply black mascara to the top and bottom lashes. If you feel confident, add single lashes and apply a creamy white pencil to the bottom inner rim of each eye.

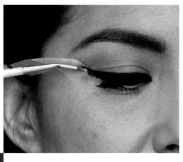

2 EYELINER

Using an eyeliner brush, apply a thick line of gel liner to the lash line. Using sticky tape as a stencil, extend to a thick taper on the outer edge of the eye, then simply remove the sticky tape to reveal a perfect line! (See also page 148.)

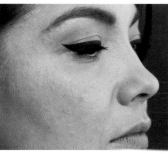

This look is great when you don't have much time.

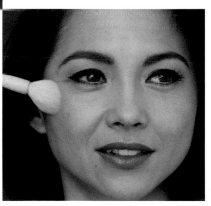

3 CHEEKS AND LIPS

Apply blush, then finish off with a lipstick in a soft mahogany shade.

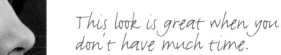

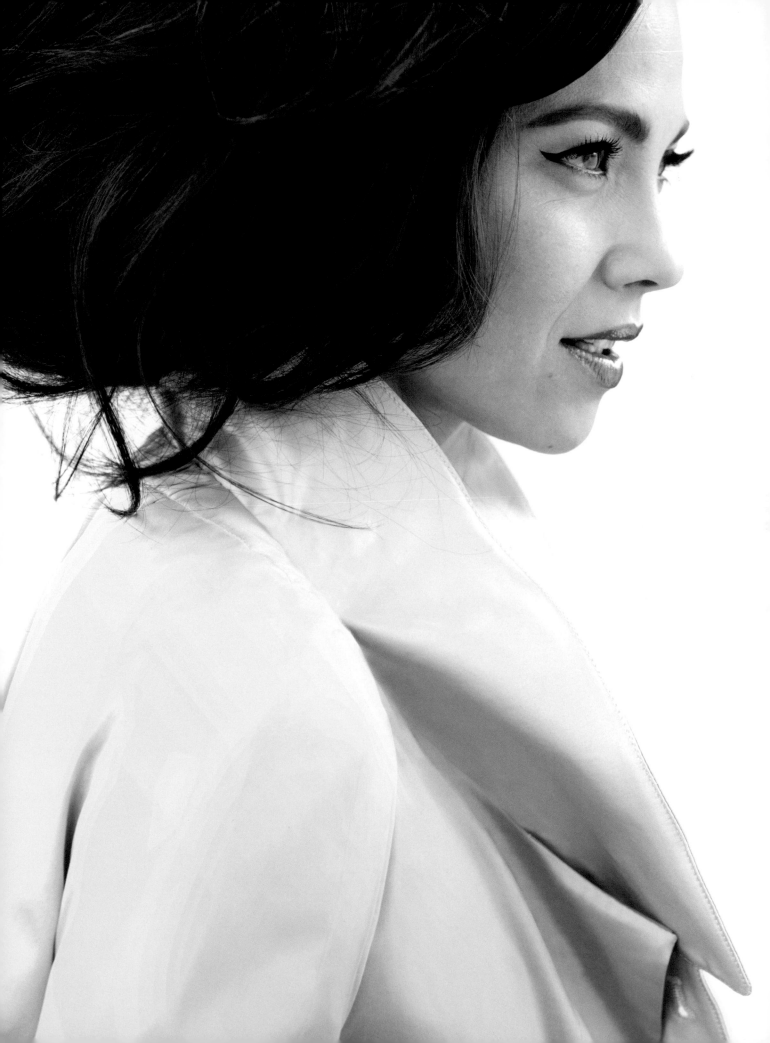

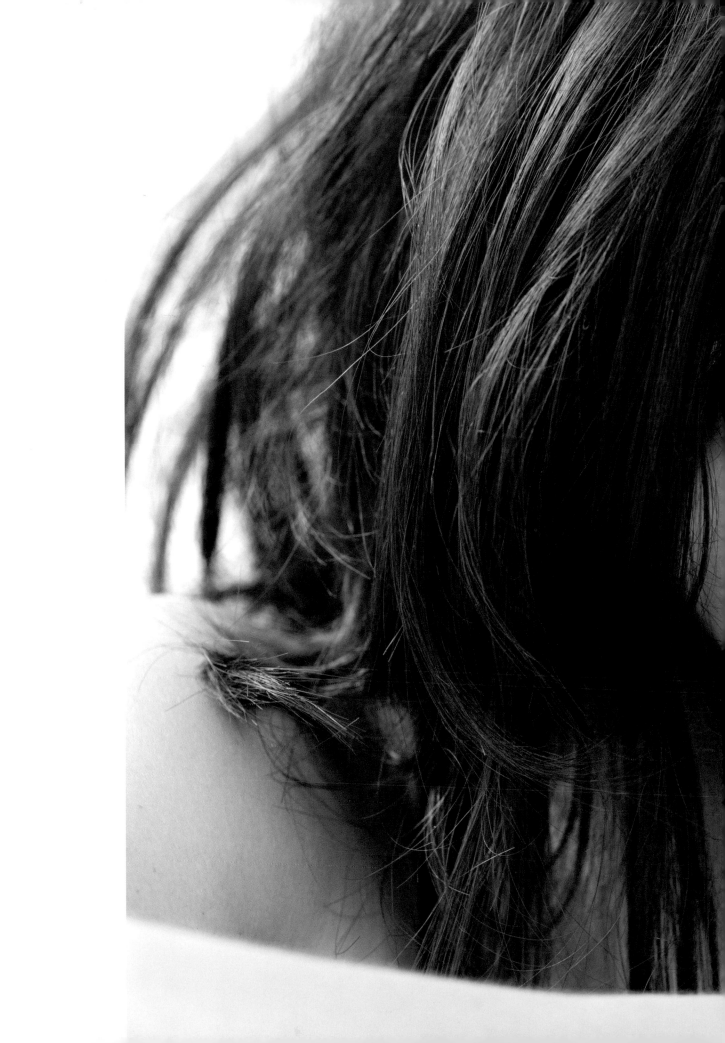

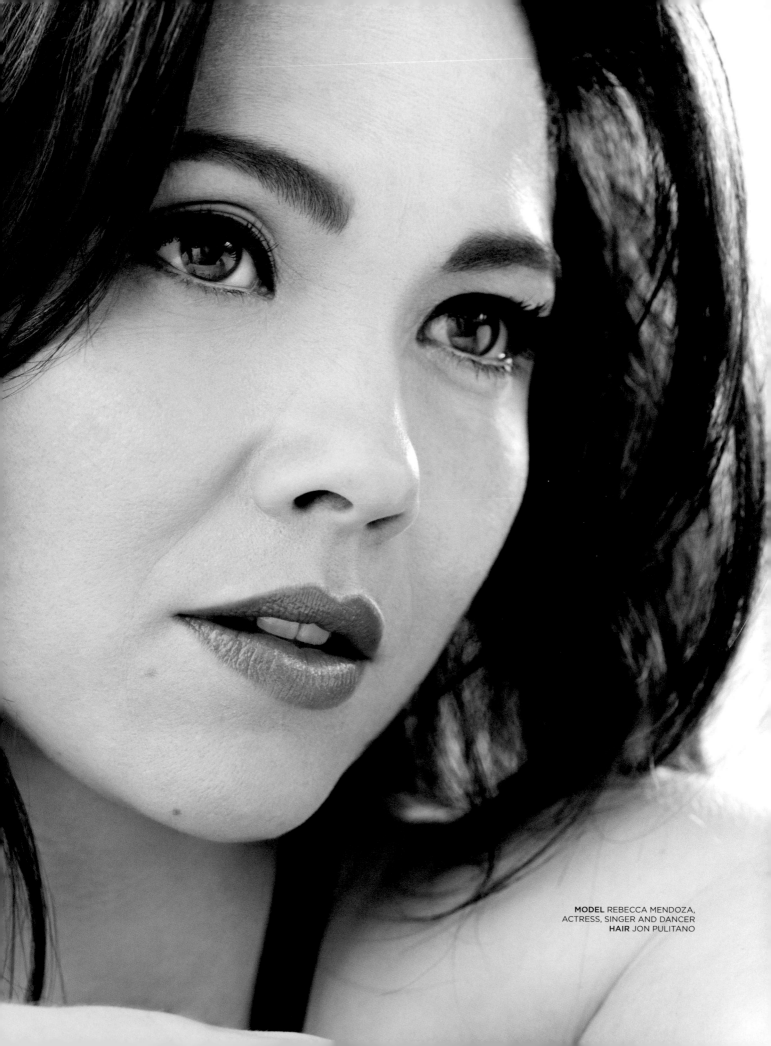

MODEL REBECCA MENDOZA,
ACTRESS, SINGER AND DANCER
HAIR JON PULITANO

Luscious Plum

HERE'S A FABULOUS WAY TO USE RICH, JEWEL-LIKE EYE SHADOWS.

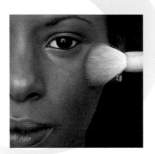

1 FOUNDATION AND POWDER

Apply foundation all over, then lightly dust the eyelids and T-zone with yellow-toned translucent powder. Dusting your T-zone will keep your skin looking ultra 'dewy'.

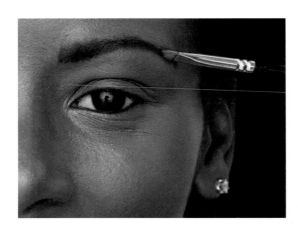

2 EYEBROWS

Define the brows. To achieve this soft line, use brow powder on an angled brush instead of a brow pencil.

3 EYE SHADOW

Apply a copper-gold eye shadow to the eyelids, and lightly contour the eye sockets with a brown matte eye shadow.

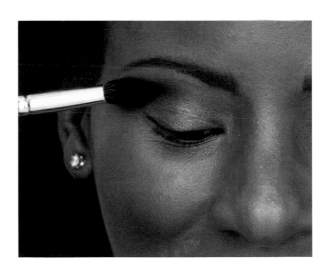

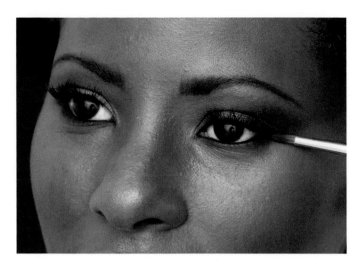

4 EYELINER AND LASHES

Smudge brown matte gel liner into the lower lash line and blend outwards. Line the inner rim with a black kohl pencil. Apply black mascara and lots of individual lashes.

5 CONTOURING AND LIPS

Apply a deep mahogany cream blush, then use a chocolate brown matte shadow to contour the nose, cheeks and forehead (see pages 34–8). Apply deep plum lipstick and finish by highlighting the cupid's bow with a copper gold shimmer.

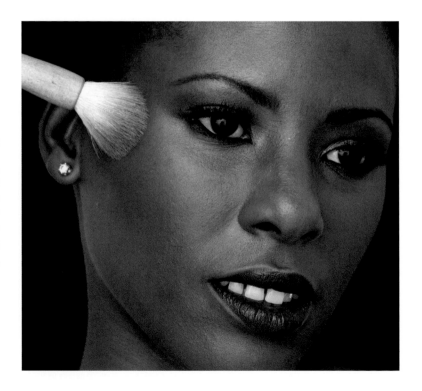

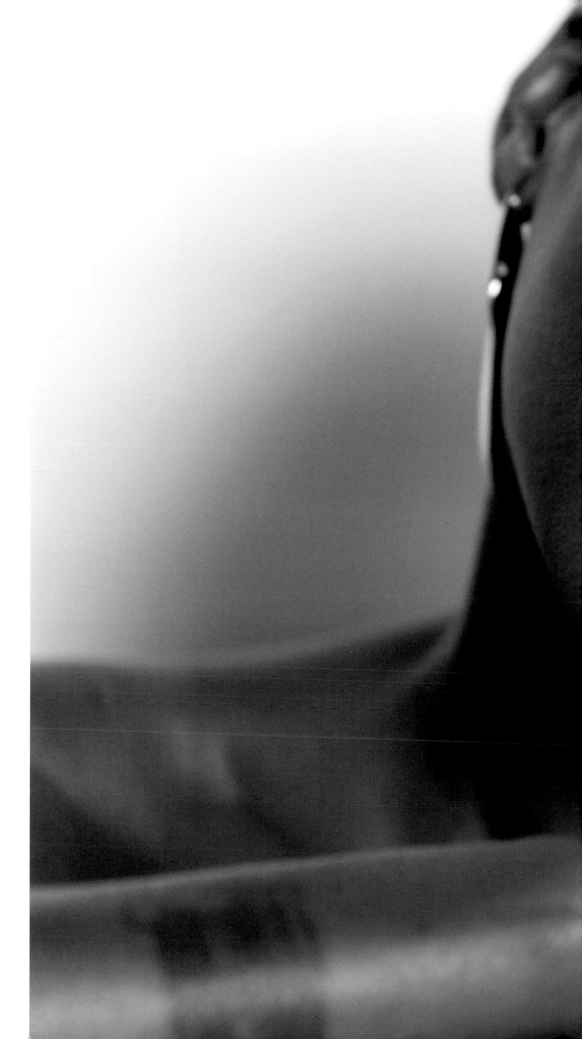

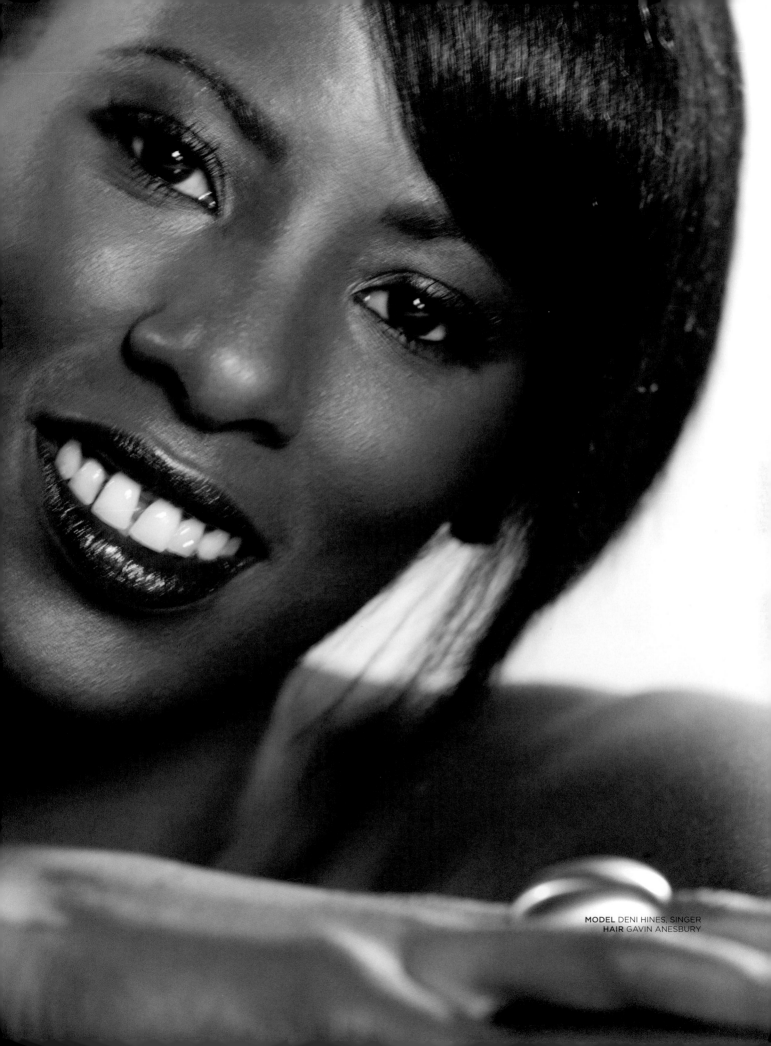

MODEL DENI HINES, SINGER
HAIR GAVIN ANESBURY

Rich Indigo

ONE INTENSE EYE SHADE IS PERFECT FOR DEWY SKIN.

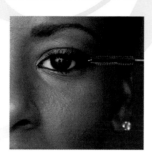

1 FOUNDATION AND EYELINER

Apply foundation all over. Lightly powder the eyelids and T-zone with yellow-toned translucent powder. Use a black kohl pencil on the eyelid to create a rectangular shape and open up the outer corner of the eye. Softly blend outwards. Apply black mascara.

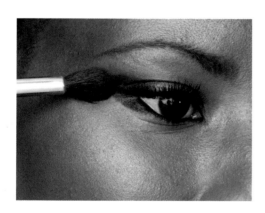

2 EYE SHADOW

Using a wet brush to avoid fallout, apply intense blue-black pigment to the eyelid and under the lower lash line. Blend while keeping the shape low and rectangular. When using a wet eye shadow, you can apply mascara first.

3 LASHES AND LIPS

Apply a 3/4 lash. Softly shade the bridge of the nose, then apply blush and a deep plum-toned lipstick. Finish with clear gloss.

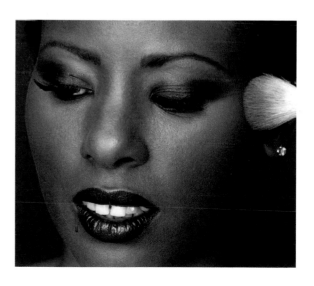

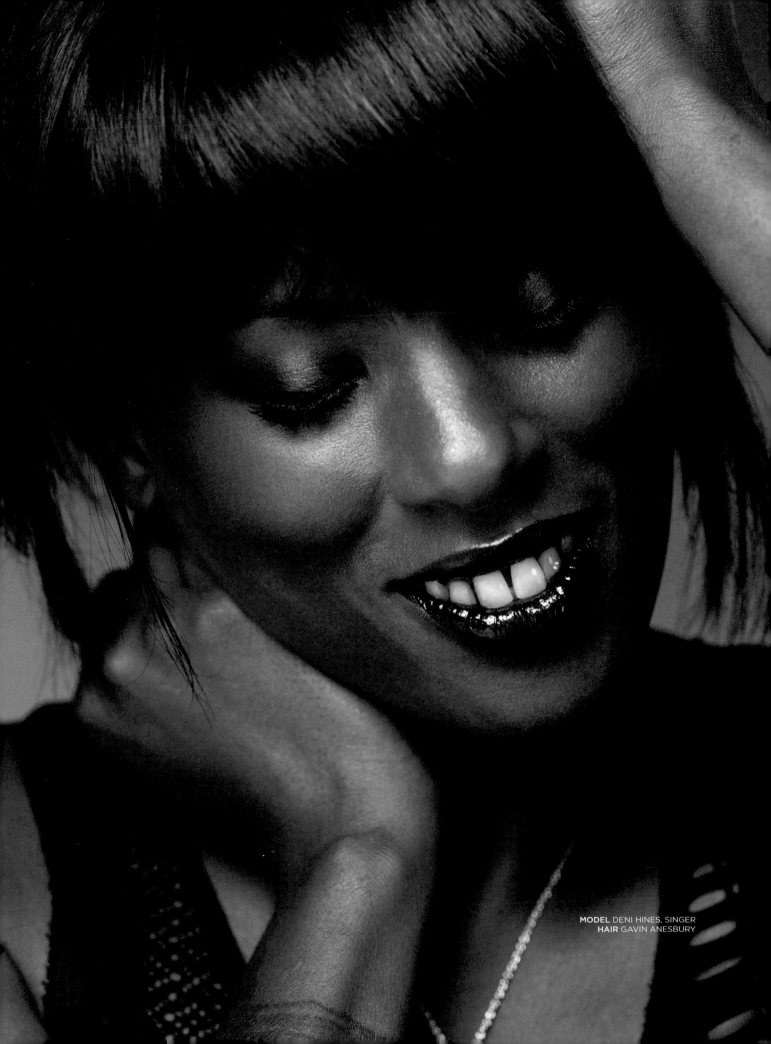

MODEL DENI HINES, SINGER
HAIR GAVIN ANESBURY

Tiger Lily

SOFTEN YOUR BROW, AND MAKE THE FOCUS THE EYE.

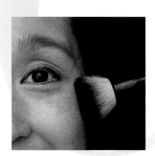

1 FOUNDATION AND EYELIDS

To disguise freckles, use a foundation brush to apply a thick cream foundation all over, buffing it into the skin so it looks sheer. To keep the skin ultra youthful, lightly powder the eyelids only with translucent powder, and apply a creamy white pencil to the inner rim of the eye.

2 EYE SHADOW, BROWS AND CHEEKS

Apply a metallic eye shadow in a coffee shade over the entire eyelid. Define the brows, and apply a pink cream blush to the cheeks.

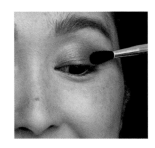

This is a good time to apply lip balm so your lips are really soft when you apply lipstick.

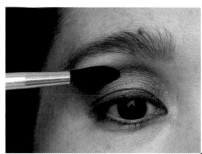

3 EYELINER AND EYE SHADOW

Apply a grey matte kohl pencil along the top and bottom outer rims of the eye. Diffuse this by blending with a lighter shade of grey eye shadow.

4 LASHES AND LIPS

Curl lashes and apply lots of black mascara. Use waterproof mascara if you prefer it. Apply single false lashes among the upper lashes only. Finish with a soft rose lipstick.

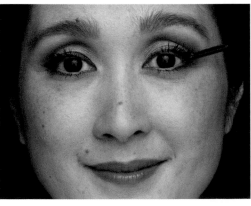

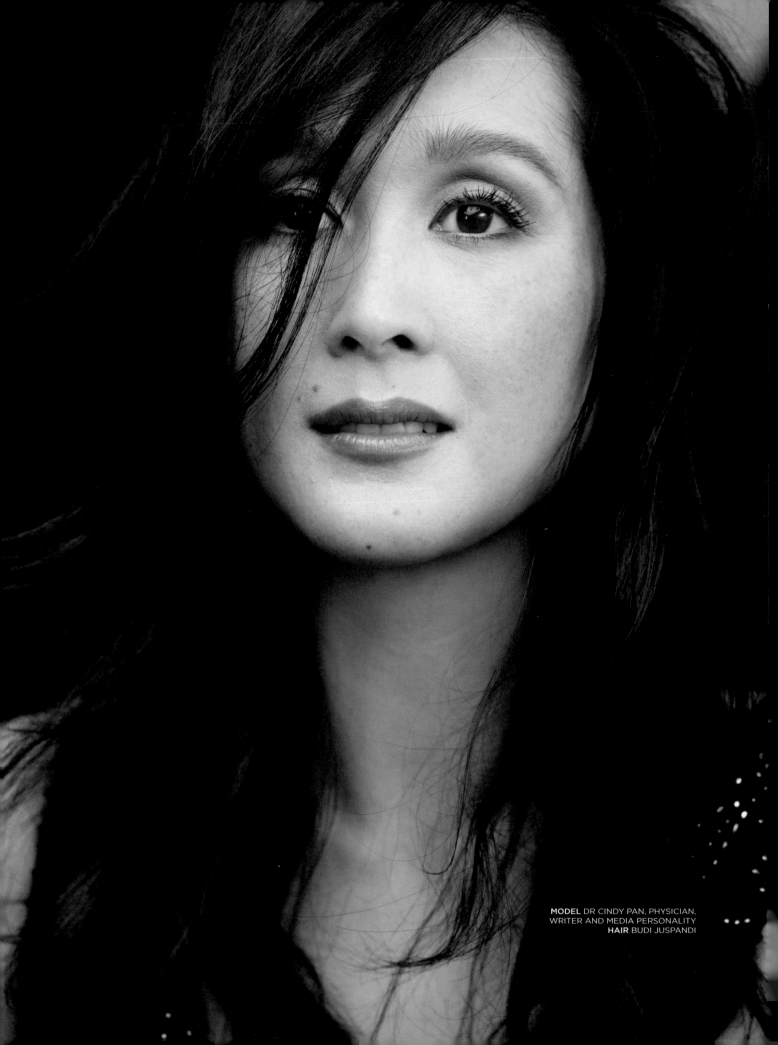

MODEL DR CINDY PAN, PHYSICIAN,
WRITER AND MEDIA PERSONALITY
HAIR BUDI JUSPANDI

Madame Butterfly

A LOOK FROM THE 1920S AND '30S THAT STILL LOOKS FABULOUS.

1 FOUNDATION AND CONCEALER

Apply a liquid foundation, then concealer where necessary.

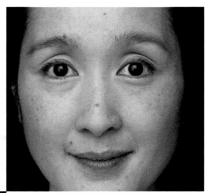

2 EYELINER

Place sticky tape on the outer edge of the eye at the desired angle. Take a black gel eyeliner and run it up the tape and along the edge of the eyelid. Peel the tape off.

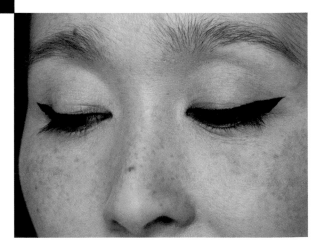

3 LASHES

Curl the lashes and apply a thick coat of waterproof black mascara. Then apply a soft full lash.

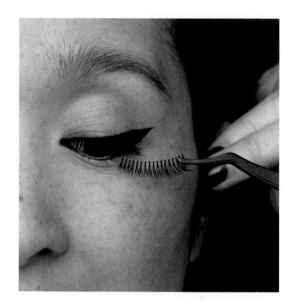

The chosen lash was a little too long, so I cut half a centimetre off the end.

4 BROWS, CONTOURING, LIPS AND HIGHLIGHTING

Define the brows, softly contour the cheeks, and apply the richest red lipstick you own. Apply a creamy white pencil to the inner lower rim of the eye. Add a soft cream gold highlight to the top of the cheekbone.

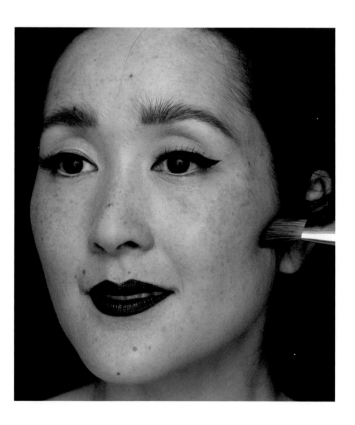

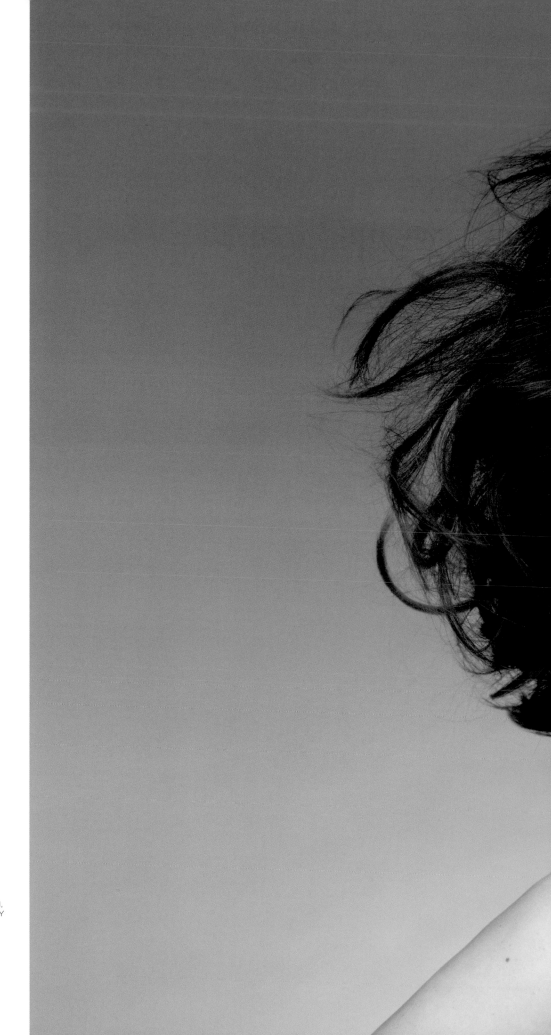

MODEL DR CINDY PAN, PHYSICIAN,
WRITER AND MEDIA PERSONALITY
HAIR GAVIN ANESBURY

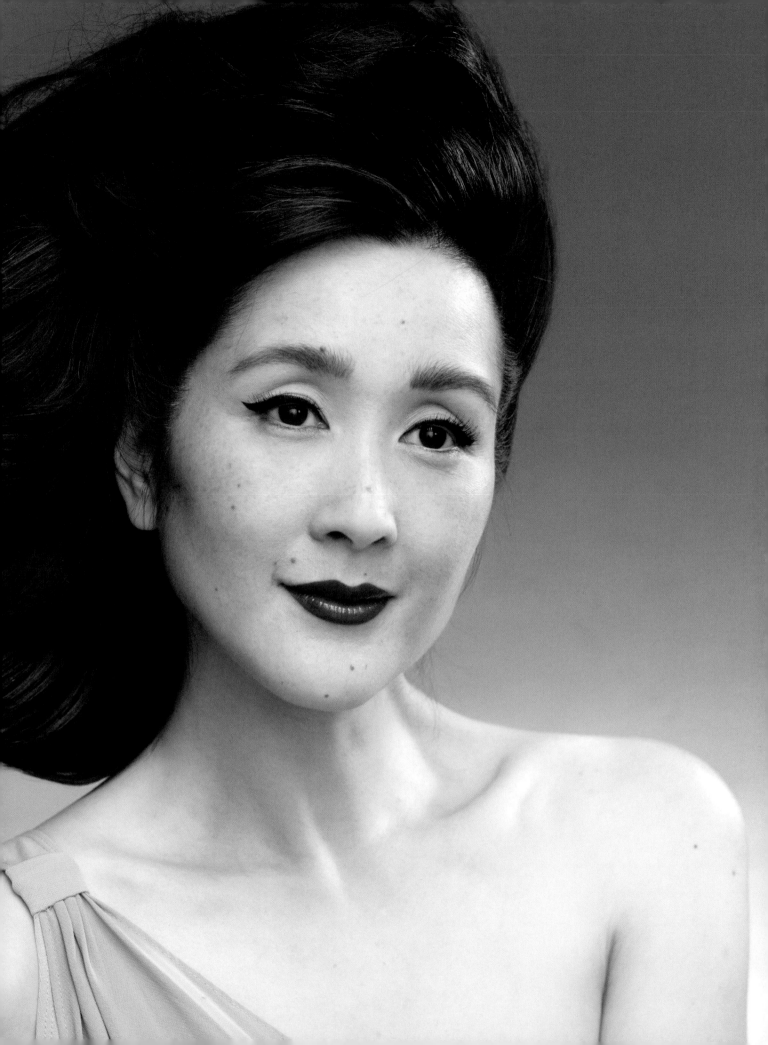

La Diva

AS THIS LOOK FEATURES SUCH A DRAMATIC EYE, I'M DOING THE EYES FIRST.

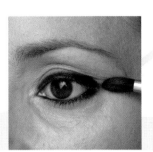

1 EYE PREP, FOUNDATION, POWDER AND EYELINER

Prep the eyes, apply foundation and lightly powder the lids only. Tina doesn't need contouring, as she has great bone structure. Use a black kohl pencil on the inner rim. Then apply a thick line along the top eyelid, blend well and extend at the outer corner.

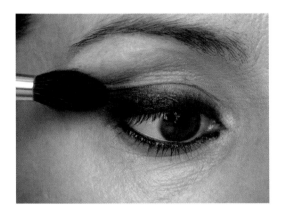

2 EYE SHADOW

Smudge a deep mahogany eye shadow along the top eyeliner and also at the outer edge of the eye to the socket line, leaving the inner area of the lid untouched.

3 EYELINER

Smudge the black kohl pencil into the outer bottom corner of the eye, keeping the shape square. This will lift the bottom of the eye, creating a more feline eye shape.

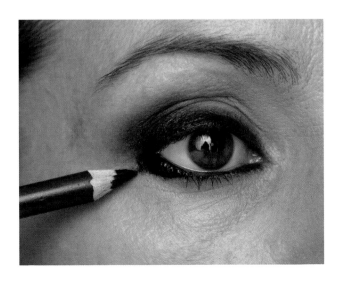

4 EYE SHADOW

Blend the deep mahogany eye shadow outwards, and try to keep the shape more square. The softer the brush pressure, the less the skin will move, cutting your blending time in half.

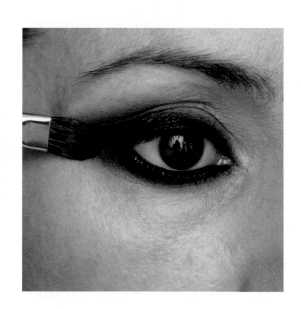

5 LASHES AND LIPS

Curl the lashes, and apply black mascara. Add just a hint of rose blush to the cheeks and some sheer rose blush to the lips.

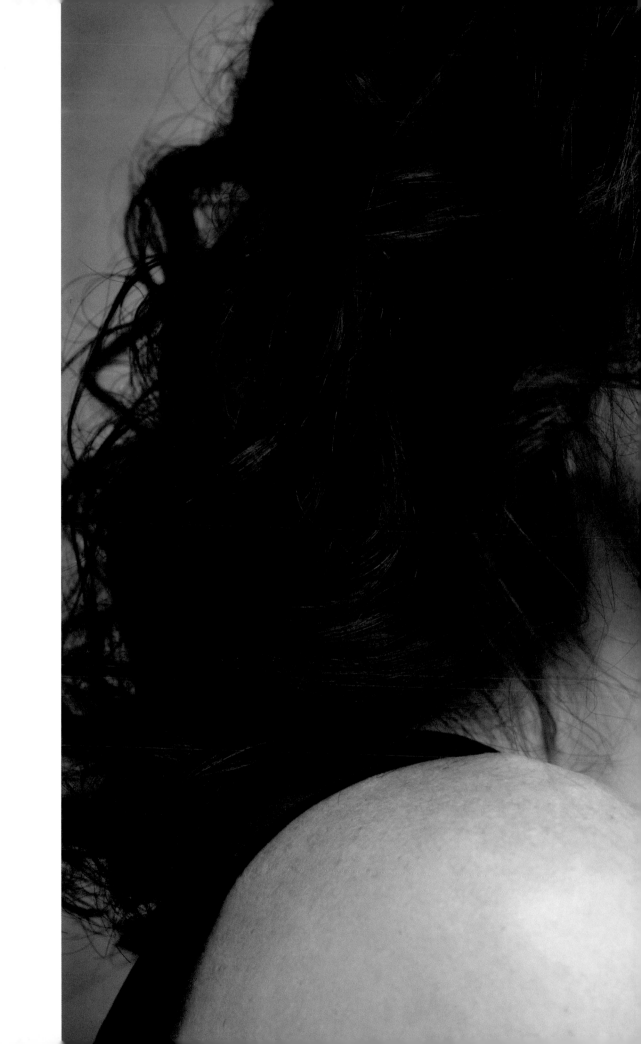

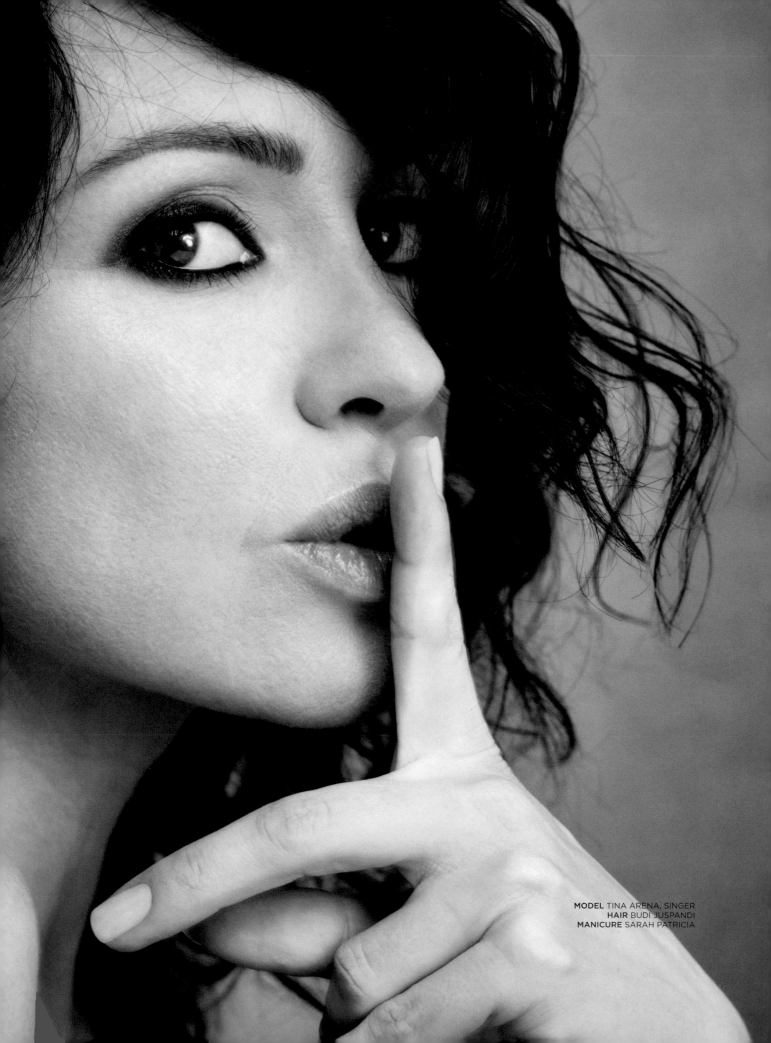

MODEL TINA ARENA, SINGER
HAIR BUDI JUSPANDI
MANICURE SARAH PATRICIA

Blonde Venus

TAKE YEARS OFF WITH THE ULTIMATE SUNKEN EYE.

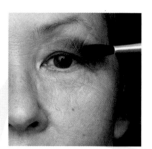

1 EYE PREP AND EYE SHADOW

Prep the eyes and apply concealer only. Apply a wash of translucent powder for optimum blending. If you have heavy eyelids like Meme, look straight ahead while applying a warm dark brown matte eye shadow over the whole lid, especially to the folding skin.

2 EYE SHADOW

To lift the eyes, apply a darker shadow on the outer lid above an imaginary line, running from the corner of the nose up to the outer corner of the eye (as shown). This area has to be the darkest point of the eye shadow.

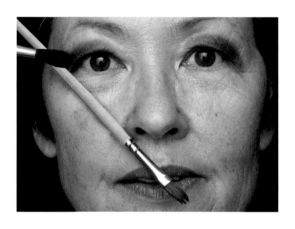

3 FOUNDATION

If, after darkening the outer corner, you feel it isn't right, or you've made a mistake, dip a clean brush in foundation or cleanser and erase anything under that same line.

4 BROWS AND FOUNDATION

Clean up any fallout under the eye. Apply foundation and concealer where necessary, and define the brows. Lowering Meme's brow arch has the effect of lifting her eye.

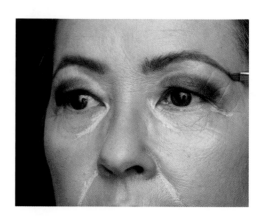

5 EYE SHADOW, BROWS AND LASHES

Use a matte light brown-golden eye shadow across the whole lid and also to soften the outer edges of dark eye shadow, then use a pencil in the same colour to do the brows. Apply a black waterproof mascara to the top lashes, then single lashes if you wish.

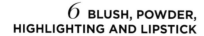

6 BLUSH, POWDER, HIGHLIGHTING AND LIPSTICK

Apply a peach cream blush. Apply powder to the T-zone or where you have excess shine. Highlight the top lip using a gold shimmer, and apply a lipstick close to your natural lip colour.

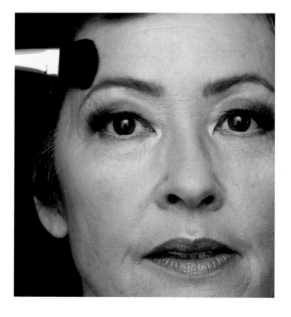

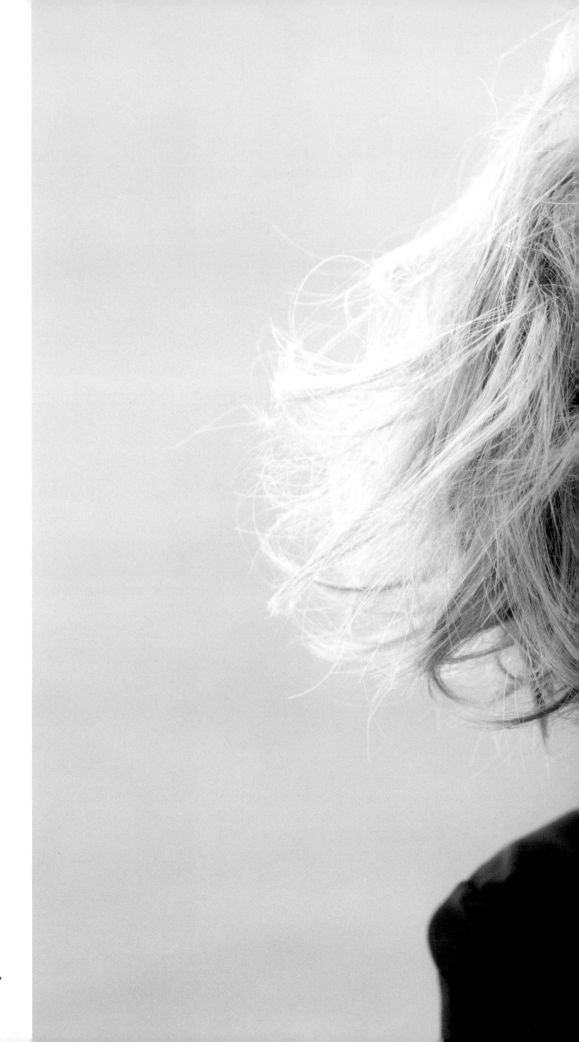

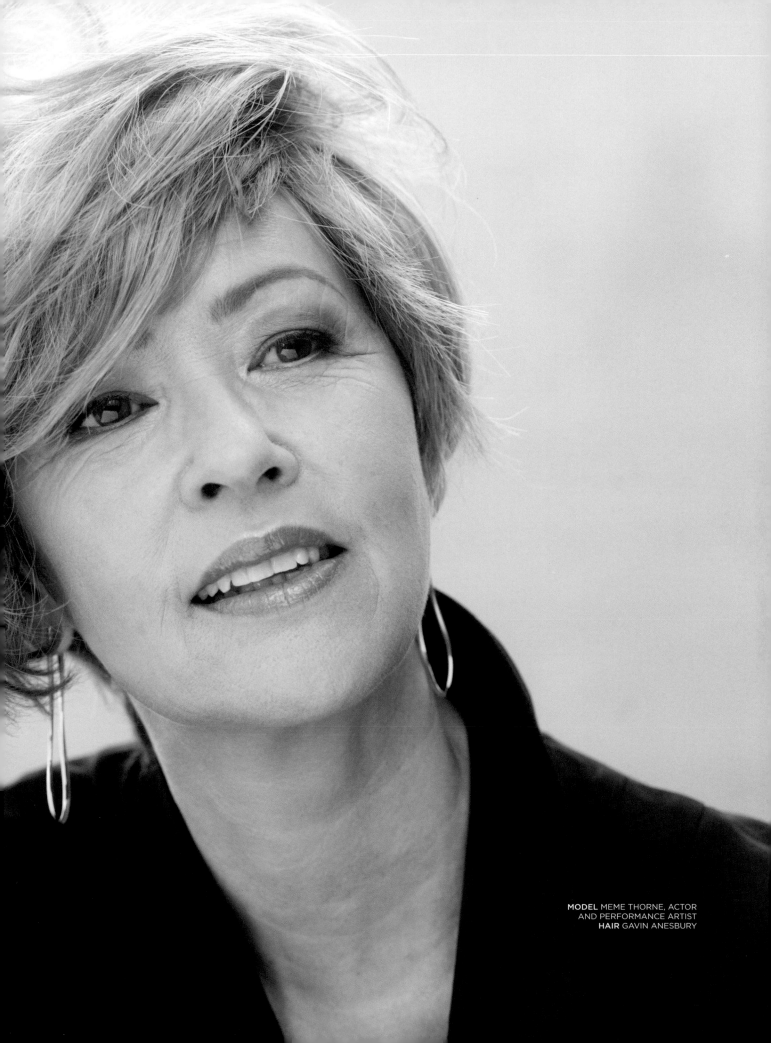

MODEL MEME THORNE, ACTOR
AND PERFORMANCE ARTIST
HAIR GAVIN ANESBURY

Beach Babe

BRONZE SHADES ARE PERFECT FOR ENHANCING A HEALTHY SUMMER GLOW.

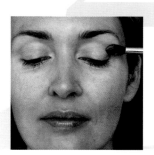

1 SKIN AND EYE PREP

Prep the skin. Because I'm applying a shimmery eye shadow—great if you have no or few lines—I'm doing the eyes first. Prep your eyes first (see page 24), then apply foundation and translucent powder to the eyelids.

2 EYE SHADOW

Apply a deep mahogany-coloured shimmery eye shadow along the lids, extending to the outer edge. You can clean up any fallout afterwards.

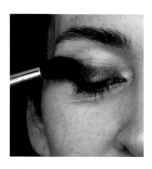

This eye shadow shade is the only colour on the colour wheel that is both cool and warm, so it will suit any skin colour or tone.

3 EYELINER AND LASHES

Apply a chocolate brown kohl pencil to the inner rim of the eye (you may need to reapply this throughout the day and evening as it fades). Then apply the kohl pencil to the outer corner of the top lid and blend well. Curl lashes and apply black mascara to the top lashes only.

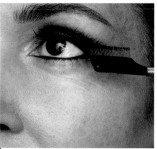

If you have dark chocolate eyes, it's best to use dark chocolate eye shadows.

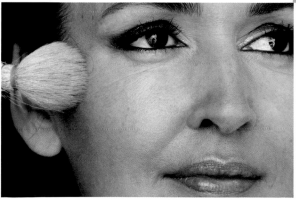

4 FOUNDATION, POWDER, BLUSH AND HIGHLIGHTING

Clean up any fallout. Apply liquid foundation, then lightly powder the T-zone if required, and apply a bronze cream blush. Choose a lip gloss that's one shade lighter than your natural lip colour. Finally, to highlight, apply gold shimmer to the inner corner of the eye and to the top of the lip.

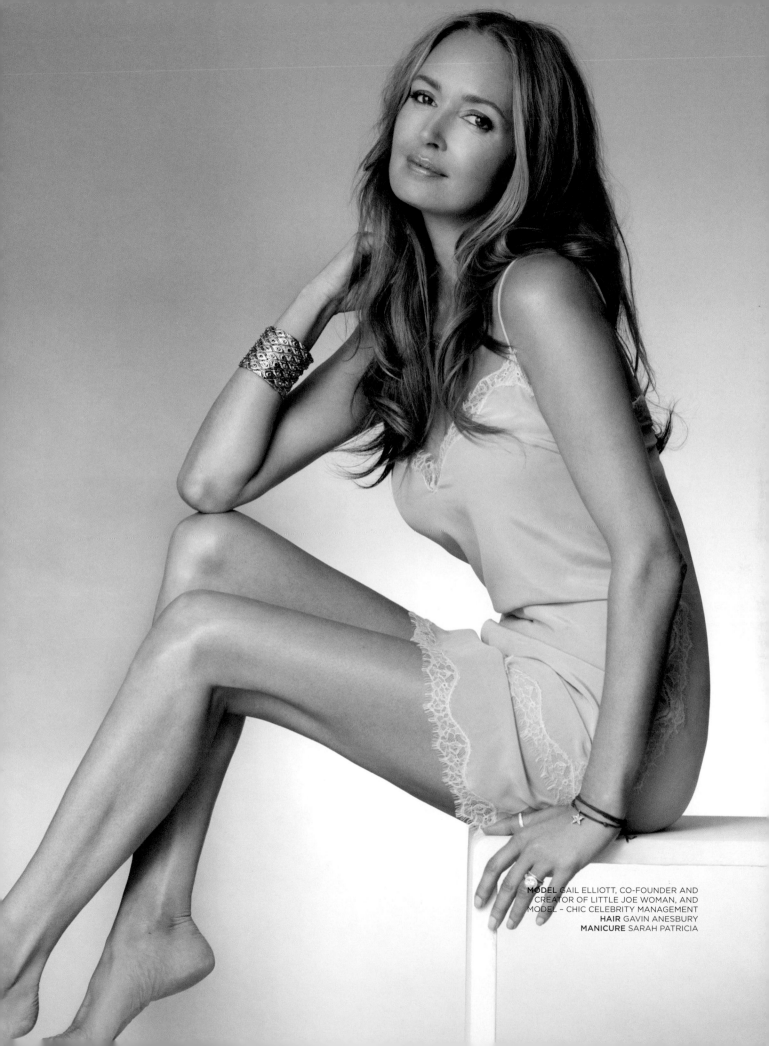

MODEL GAIL ELLIOTT, CO-FOUNDER AND
CREATOR OF LITTLE JOE WOMAN, AND
MODEL – CHIC CELEBRITY MANAGEMENT
HAIR GAVIN ANESBURY
MANICURE SARAH PATRICIA

Evening Star

A HOT CORPORATE LOOK. SIMPLY ADD A GLAMOROUS DRESS FOR NIGHT.

1 SKIN AND EYE PREP

Use a foundation brush to apply liquid foundation in a very warm, golden shade all over, then concealer where necessary.

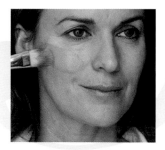

Make sure you also apply foundation to your neck, which may be slightly paler than your face and chest.

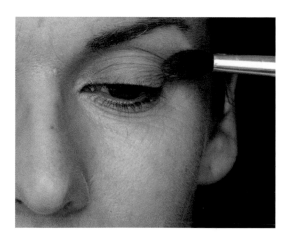

2 CONTOURING

Shade and contour the cheeks and eyes (see pages 35 and 37). Smooth out any foundation lines on the eyelids, and lightly powder.

3 BROWS AND EYELINER

Define your brows, lowering the arch if necessary. Apply black gel eyeliner into the top lash line (right along the lash bed) to define.

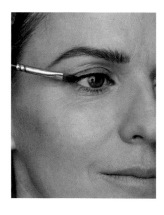

When applying eyeliner to the bottom lash line, make your eyes look bigger by picking the lowest point on the bottom of the eye and shading along a slightly straight line rather than the natural curve. I rarely join bottom and top eyeliner, especially on round eyes.

4 EYE SHADOW

While looking straight ahead into the mirror, use a grey matte eye shadow to shade the outer corner of the lid, which you most want to push back.

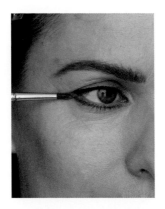

Keep a clean brush with translucent powder on standby for blending and softening. The lighter the pressure of the brush, the less the skin moves, which results in better blending.

5 LASHES

Curl your lashes, and apply black mascara to the top and bottom lashes. Apply single lashes in any gaps along the upper lash line.

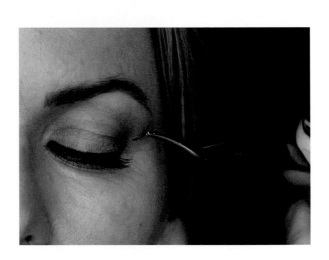

6 BLUSH, HIGHLIGHTING AND LIPSTICK

If your skin tends to be shiny, blot with blotting papers throughout the day, or use a translucent powder to take away the shine. Apply cream blush, then highlight the cupid's bow with gold shimmer powder. Finish off with a soft pink lipstick.

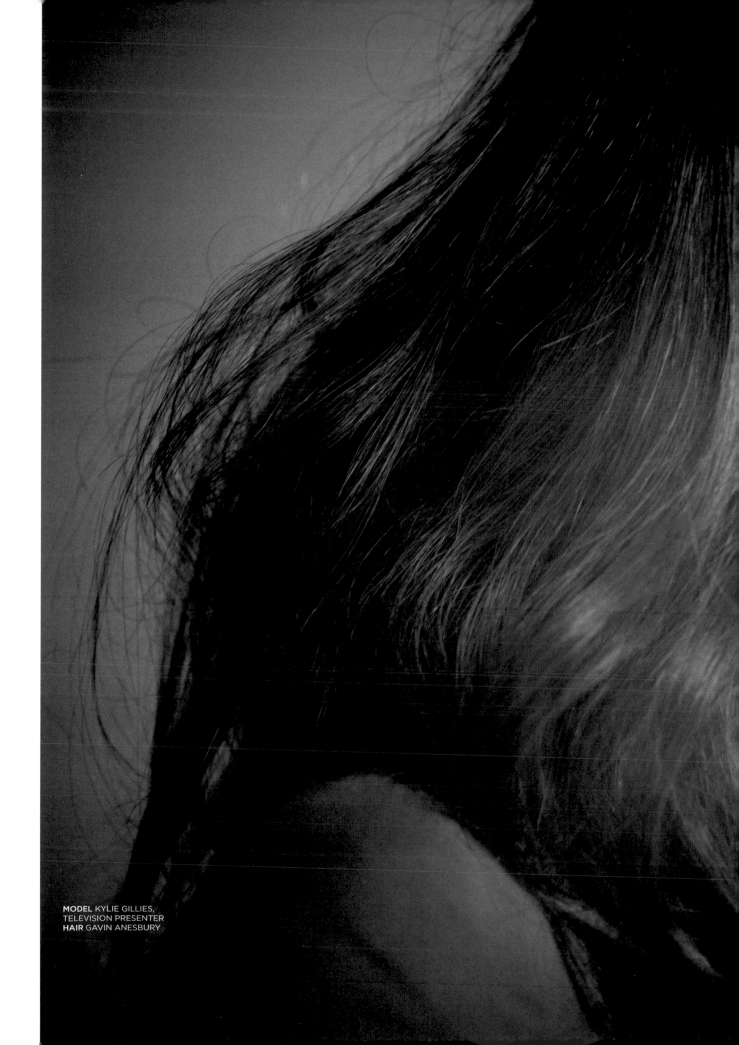

MODEL KYLIE GILLIES,
TELEVISION PRESENTER
HAIR GAVIN ANESBURY

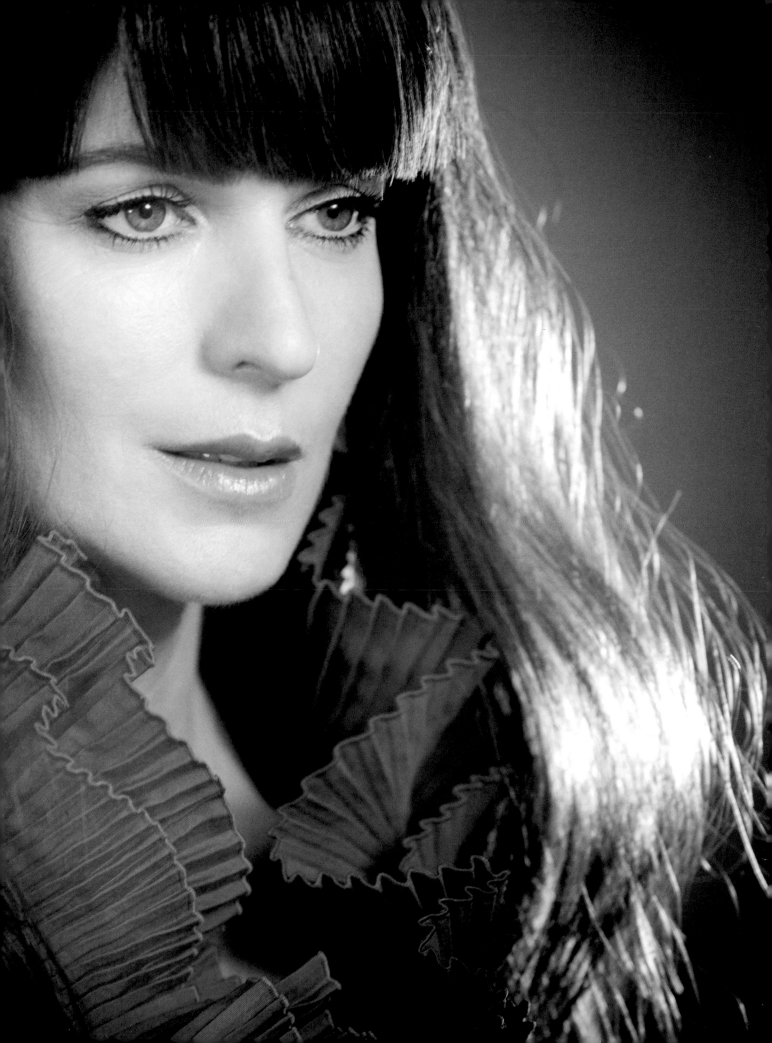

Wild Orchid

IF YOU'RE OBSESSED WITH COLOUR, THIS LOOK IS FOR YOU.

1 SKIN PREP AND EYE SHADOW

Prep your skin, and remove any oil from your eyelids. Next, apply foundation to your eyelids only, then powder them with translucent powder. Apply intense violet eye shadow and lip balm.

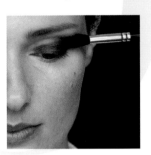

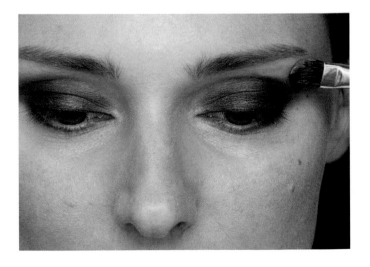

2 EYELINER AND EYE SHADOW

Apply a deep violet gel eyeliner along the top lash line and blend it into the eyelash bed. Lightly conceal under the eye, and apply a soft wash of matte violet eye shadow along the bottom lash line.

3 INNER RIMS AND EYE SHADOW

Use a creamy white pencil on the inner rims, then a larger blending brush and translucent powder to softly blend the eye shadow.

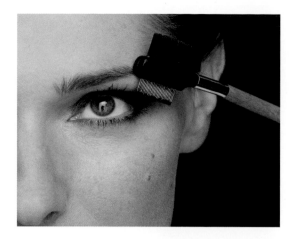

4 FOUNDATION, POWDER AND MASCARA

Clean up the fall-out, apply foundation, conceal where necessary and set with powder. Apply loads of black mascara to both the top and bottom lashes.

5 EYEBROWS

Groom the eyebrows. I've lowered the arch of Anneliese's brows, lifting her eyes more. This brow shape is one of my favourites.

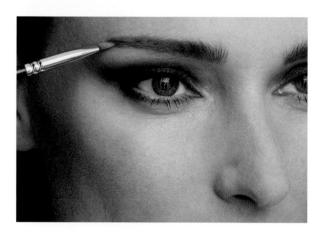

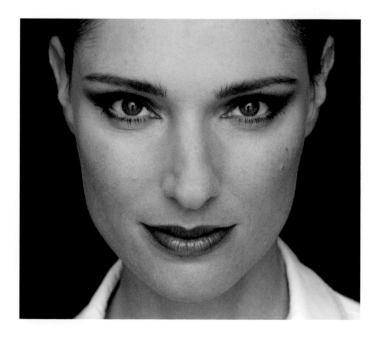

6 LIPS

Finally, apply a bright red-mahogany lipstick.

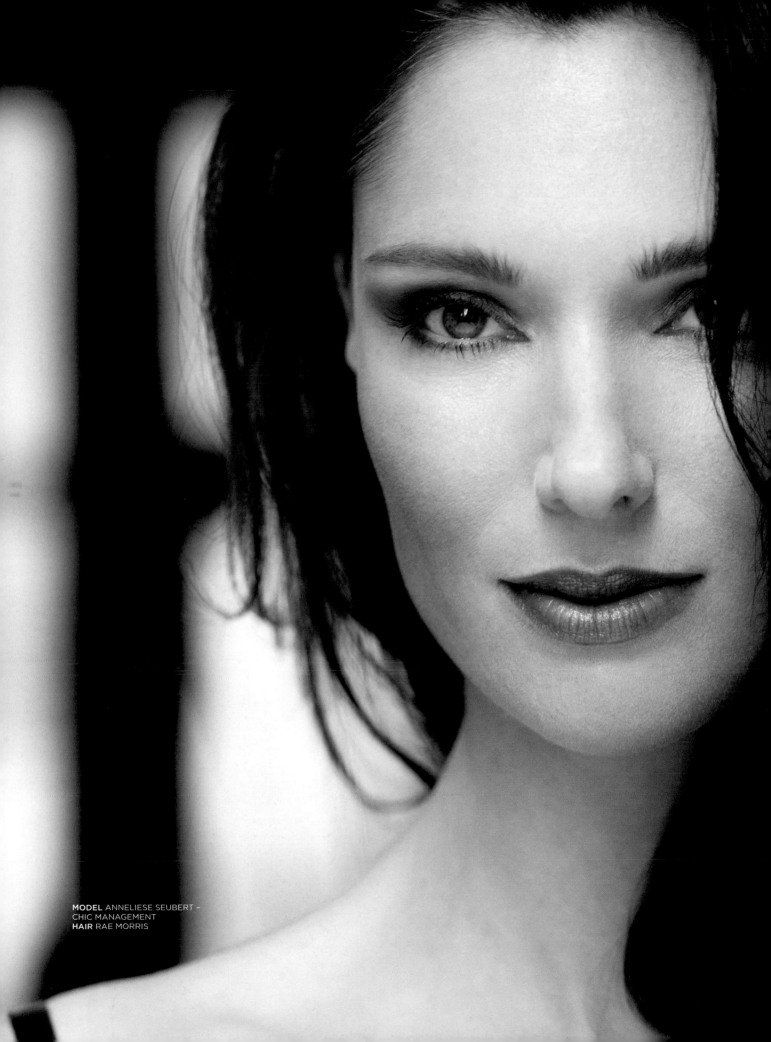

MODEL ANNELIESE SEUBERT –
CHIC MANAGEMENT
HAIR RAE MORRIS

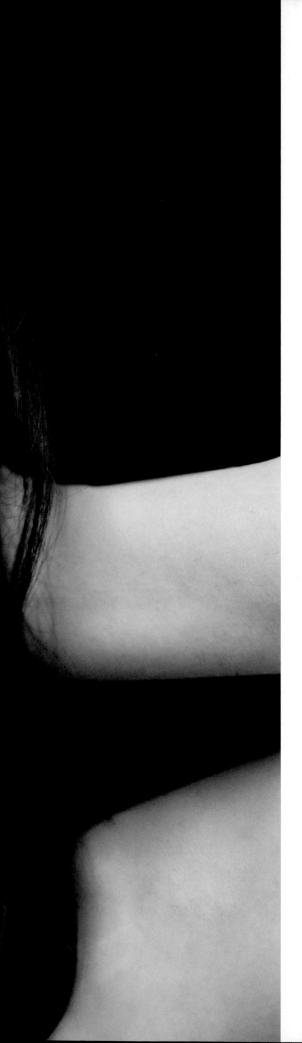

Non-surgical cosmetic techniques

Alternatives to makeup—such as botox, laser treatments and fillers—can be a touchy subject, but cosmetic enhancements have become part of day-to-day life.

There are some amazing non-invasive techniques, which have their place, depending on what you are trying to achieve. By non-invasive techniques I mean there is no actual surgery involved. For example, did you know that one small injection can instantly remove dark circles from under your eyes? I have even seen broken capillaries disappear within twenty-four hours of laser treatment.

First, let me say that I love lines—they add character, tell your story and help make you who you are. Some of the most beautiful images in the world are of women who have aged gracefully and naturally, and bring their own unique qualities into the shot. Leona Edmiston is one of those beautiful women.

But if you're spending hundreds of dollars on skincare and cosmetics that claim to hide and reduce lines, not to mention the time you spend applying them every day, then you might want to consider paying for instant results a couple of times a year.

Most of the middle-aged women you see on the red carpet have had 'something' done, even if it is subtle. You'll only notice if it's been done badly. If you've undergone a non-surgical technique, you should look glowing and refreshed, as if you've been on holiday—any lines should just be softened and subtle. If it's noticeable for the wrong reasons, it's too much.

You have to put the idea of non-surgical techniques into your own personal context—there is no one solution that fits all. It's a matter of what will make you look better and help you feel more confident. My advice is to keep it looking natural.

Some common problems can now be corrected instantly and non-invasively. These include: smokers' lines around the mouth; baggy eyes; heavy, hooded brows; droopy eyes; and dull, aged skin. Non-invasive techniques can even soften jowls, re-create jaw lines, correct hollowing (for example, at the temples and under the eyes) and enhance cheeks.

I keep up to date with the latest cosmetic techniques by regularly consulting a cosmetic doctor. I won't list all the current procedures because this area is constantly evolving, and by the time you read this, even more amazing procedures will be available.

If you want to head down the path of non-invasive cosmetic enhancement techniques, thoroughly research the particular treatments you're interested in, then arrange a consultation with a reputable cosmetic doctor who can tailor the procedures to suit you.

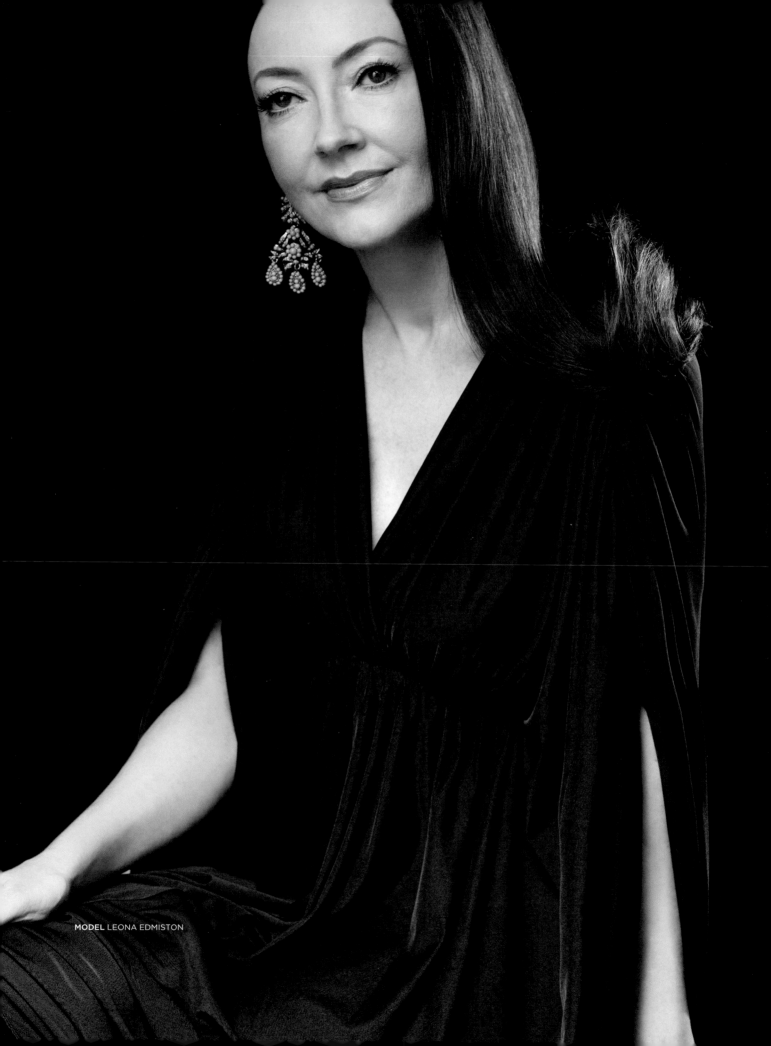

MODEL LEONA EDMISTON

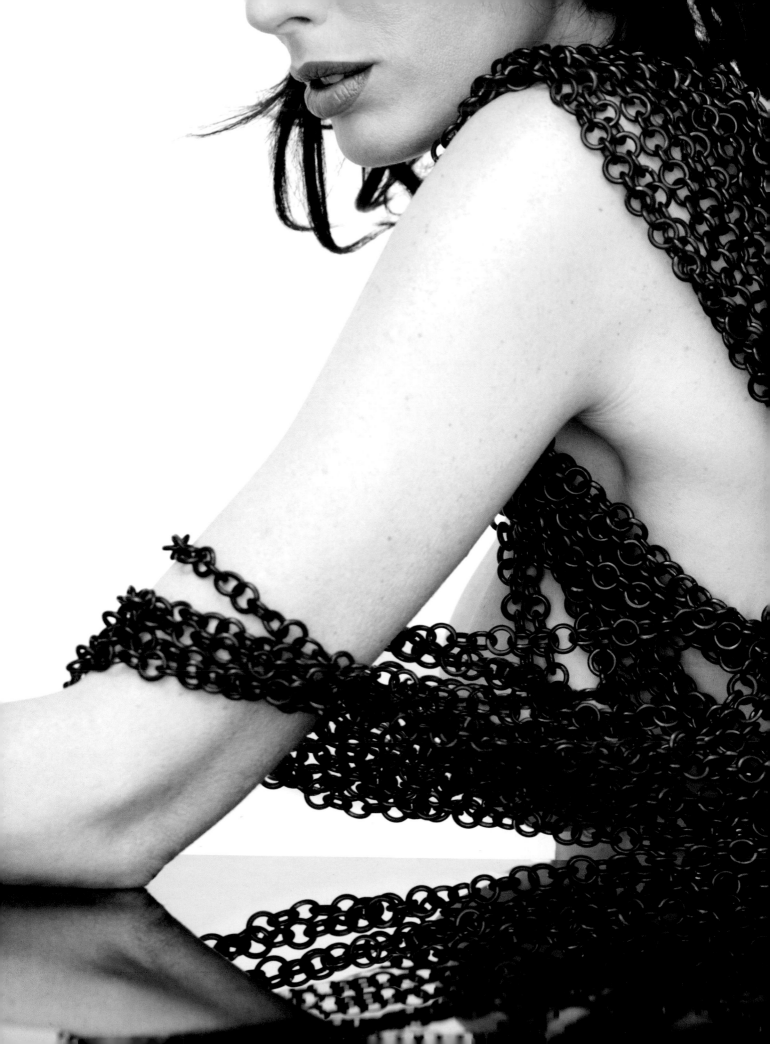

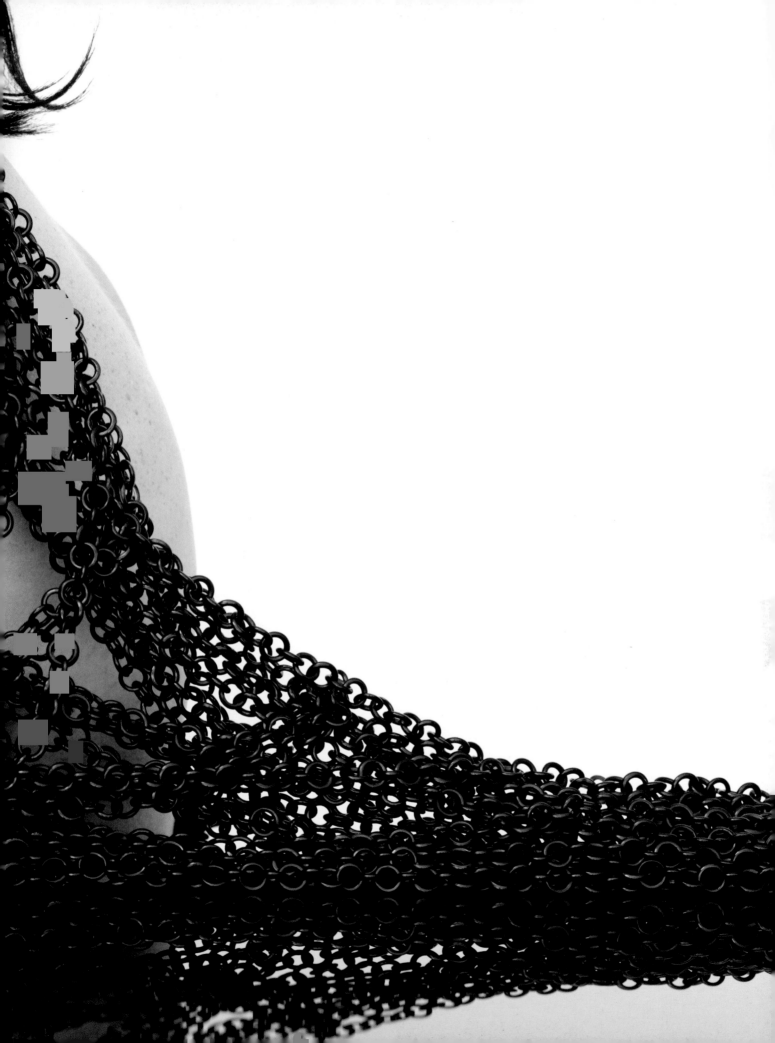

Index

Page numbers in *italics* refer to photographs

eyelashes
  ageing &, 5
  extensions for, 5, 43
  false, 43, 62–4, *62, 63, 64, 65–7*, 91, *91*
  length of, 43
  see also Looks
eyelid ageing, 4, 37, 42, 43
eyelid moisturisation, 27
eyeliner, 5, 19, *19*, 79
  see also Looks
eyeliner brushes, 13, *13*
eyes
  ageing of, 4, 5, 42, 54, 170
  close-set, 43
  contouring &, 37, *37, 39*, 107, *107,
    162, 162*
  non-surgical cosmetic techniques
    for, 170
  prescription glasses &, 78
  shape enhancement &, 42, 43, *43*
  size of, 43

F

face and body scrub, 11, 27
face powder
  ageing &, 5
  full makeup kit, 16
  see also Looks; translucent powder
fallout, 102, *102*
false eyelash applicators, 62, *63*, 64,
  64, 91
false eyelashes, 43, 62–4, *63, 64, 65,
  91, 91*
  see also individual lashes
fan brush, 15, *15*
feet, 27

forehead, high, 36, *36*
foundation
  ageing &, 5, 27
  full-makeup kit, 16
  glasses frames &, 79
  lips &, 71, 73
  skin texture &, 29–31, *29, 30, 31*
  touch-up kit, 10
  types of, 16, 28, 29–31
  see also Looks
foundation brushes, 12, *12*
freckles, 146
French Marigold look, 112–13, *112, 113,
  114–15*
full-makeup kits, 11–21

G

glasses frames, 78–81, 79, *80–1*
gold highlighter, 17, 163
green eye colour charts, 50–1, *50–1*
green eye look, 102–3, *102, 103, 104–5*
Green Ice look, 96–7, *96, 97, 98–9*

H

hair, 77
hairline contouring, 36, *36*, 90, *90*, 103,
  113, 117, 120
hand cream, 10
hands, 4, 5, 27
hazel eye colour charts, 52–3, *52–3*
highlighters, 17, *17*
highlighting, 133, *133*, 157, 160, 163
Honeysuckle Rose look, 102–3, *102, 103,
  104–5*

I

individual lashes, 43, 62, *66*, 110, *110*, 146,
  163, *163*
intensifying eye shadow colours, 46–53,
  46–53

J

jaw line, 4, 36
jewellery, 5, 70, 71, 76

K

kabuki brush, 14, *14*, 113, *113*
kohl pencils, 19, *19*, 94, 102, 141, 144, 146,
  152, 160

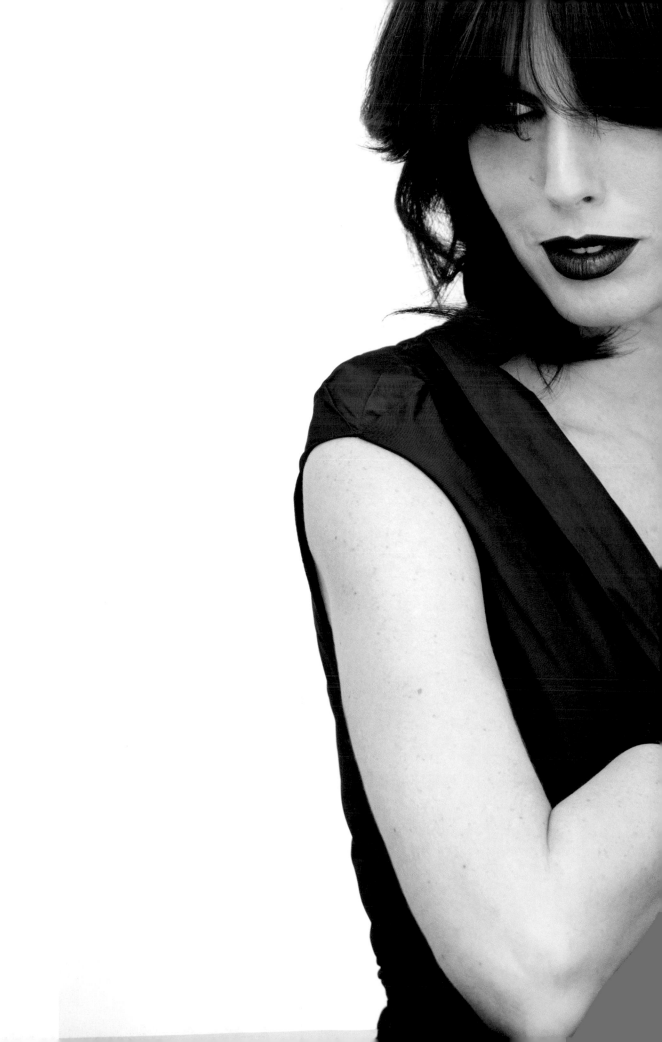

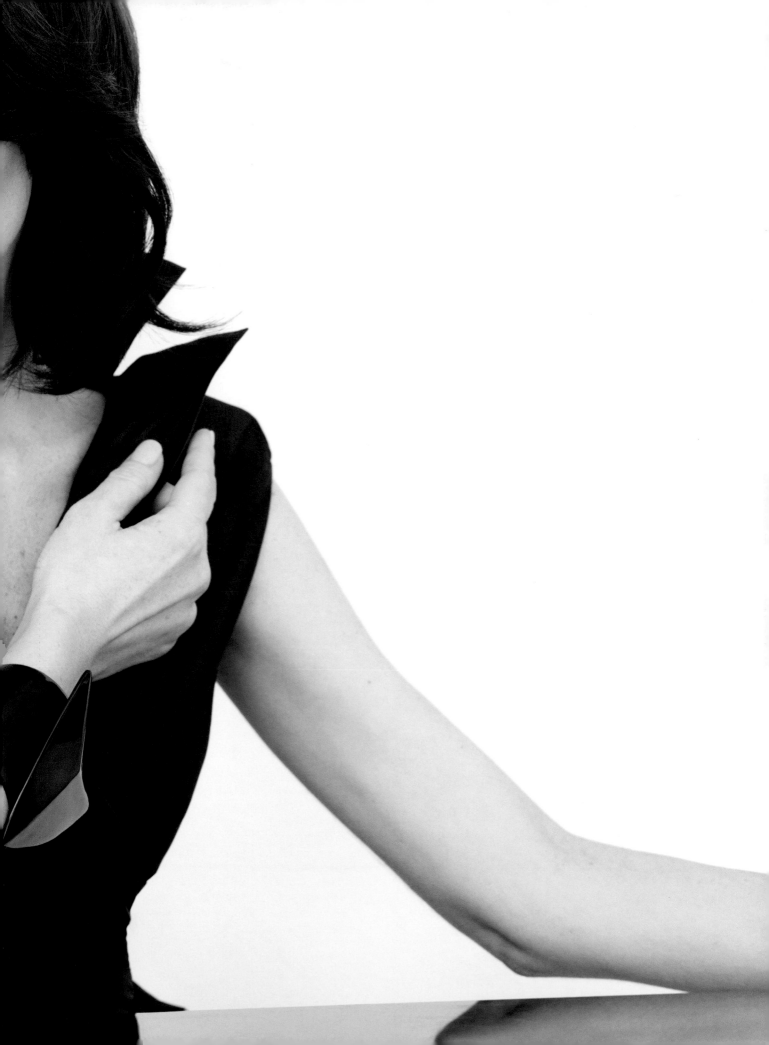

Acknowledgments

Jason Capobianco—our amazing photographer. Not only have you supported me from the beginning of my career but you also patiently held my hand and guided me through each and every shot in this book. You came in every day with a smile on your face and, with such professionalism, made all these women feel so comfortable in front of the camera. And yes, they are all still talking about you!

Jason's amazing team—Anton Perry, Romello Pereira, Kylie Coutts, James Green, Bec Howell and Jason Sievers.

My wonderful assistants—Lei Tai, Priscilla Rasjid, Casey Gore and Ashley Penfold. I could not do my job without you. You were there 'early' every day, even Sundays! Thank you for always thinking one step ahead of me and for your inexhaustible enthusiasm—you made this project fun and definitely memorable!

Grace Testa (www.gracetesta.com), our talented retoucher. This is our third book together and with every shot we took I had complete confidence that the end result would match the beauty we saw in real life.

My manicurist Sarah Patricia Todd (www.sarahpatricia.com.au). You were there until the end of each day, pampering my models. Such perfection, toes and all!

All the amazing women who gave up their time to be photographed for this book. You were all wonderful and incredibly beautiful, and you let me just do my thing. The shots in this book go beyond beauty—you gave them heart, soul and personality, the sort of depth that takes life experience. I never wanted the shoots to end. A special thanks to Tina Arena, who turned up after a sleepless flight from Paris and gave one hundred per cent.

Julie Anderson—what a superstar you are. You grace the cover and all the title pages. You made us laugh, and blew us all away with your beauty, your body and the fact that you are—yes—forty years old!

Jon Pulitano at Headcase Hair, Gavin Anesbury and Budi Juspandi, our divine and talented hair stylists, for the styles you created and the way you made all the women feel and look so beautiful.

Our stylist Emma Wood, who dressed these women and devoted her time to this project, and Alistair Trung, Carla Zampatti and Bunda Jewellery for their support.

Alistair Trung, the amazing designer, for going the extra mile. Alistair, I just had to have your clothes on the cover.

Bronwyn Fraser, whose colour guides appeared first in *Makeup: The Ulimate Guide* and stand up to this day.

Nanette Cornish, who read and reread transcripts and helped fine tune the text, and my assistant Erinn Vassilimis, who proofread the finished book.

David Ryrie at S2 Studios, for the use of their amazing studio and making us feel at home everyday. It didn't feel like work.

Louise Thurtell, my publisher at Allen & Unwin, and Sarah Baker, my editor. How can I thank you? Your patience with me yet again was just outstanding. You have no idea how essential both your support and advice has been to me. You make me want to write more books, and you were a big part of my inspiration for this one.

Robert Gorman, CEO of Allen & Unwin, for his commitment to health and beauty, and for being such a huge supporter of my books.

Stephen Smedley, of Tonto Design, who designed this book. Steve, it was so easy. You just kept getting it right!

Lisa Farrow and Reload Agency, who tirelessly support me not only in this but in everything I do. Lisa, you are always there—you have been at every launch, every book press day. You're the best agent I've ever had. Thank you! You go way beyond the call of duty.

Mark Byrne, my literary agent. You made the dream come alive. Who would have predicted a 'trilogy'!

Maree Mitchell, of Title Artist Management, who pulled all this together.

Trinny and Susannah. Even after all my years in this industry, you have taught me so much. Throughout this book are pieces inspired by you. Trinny, thank you for such a beautiful foreword—I'm truly touched.

Jim Cornish, I had to save you until the end. I could not have done this without you. As you know, this book was a 24/7 obsession. Thank you for all the tireless nights you listened to me and helped me write. You are my walking thesaurus, and no one can translate 'Rae' like you.

CREDITS

Cover and vi Top by Alistair Trung.

viii and 108–9 Denim jacket by Diesel. Earrings by Erikson Beamon.

2–3 and 101 Hair – Jon Pulitano. Manicure – Sarah Patricia. Lingerie – Obsidian by Elle Macpherson Intimates.

7 and 161 Silk slip by Little Joe. Jewellery model's own.

8–9 Hair – Gavin Anesbury. Manicure – Sarah Patricia. Dress by Bettina Liano. Jewellery by Bunda.

22–3 Hair – Jon Pulitano. Manicure – Sarah Patricia. Top by Alistair Trung.

32–3 Hair – Gavin Anesbury. Manicure – Sarah Patricia. Jewellery by Alistair Trung.

40–1 Hair – Jon Pulitano. Manicure – Sarah Patricia. Hat by American Apparel. Dress by Zimmerman. Vintage jewellery.

68–9 Hair – Jon Pulitano. Manicure – Sarah Patricia. Jewellery by Alistair Trung.

74–5 Hair – Gavin Anesbury.

77 Shirt by Jac & Jack.

79–81 Selection of glasses by Paul Taylor, Tom Ford and Dsquared.

82–3 Hair – Gavin Anesbury. Manicure – Sarah Patricia. Dress by Bettina Liano.

88–9 Jacket by Carla Zampatti.

92–3 Vintage Gucci jacket.

95 Top by Bettina Liano.

98–9 Top by Jac & Jack. Jewellery by Bunda.

104–5 Shirt by Sportscraft. Jewellery by Bunda.

111 Dress by Alistair Trung.

114–15 Top by Jac & Jack. Jeans by J Brand. Cuff by Mania Mania. Earrings by Paul & Joe.

118–19 Top by No-lita. Jeans by J Brand. Vintage earrings.

121 Annalise Signature Lingerie and Jewellery. Hoodie by Bonds.

125 Jacket by Carla Zampatti. Necklace by Bunda.

126–7 Jacket by Carla Zampatti.

129 and 170 Dress by Leona Edmiston. Earrings model's own.

131 Top by Alistair Trung. Jeans by J Brand.

137 Vintage Scanlan & Theodore jacket.

142–3 Jewellery by Bunda.

145 Top by No-lita. Jewellery by Bunda.

158–9 Jewellery by Bunda.

164–5 Jacket by Giorgio Armani.

172–3 Chains by Alistair Trung.

178–9 Hair – Jon Pulitano. Manicure – Sarah Patricia. Jacket by Carla Zampatti. Jewellery by Alistair Trung.

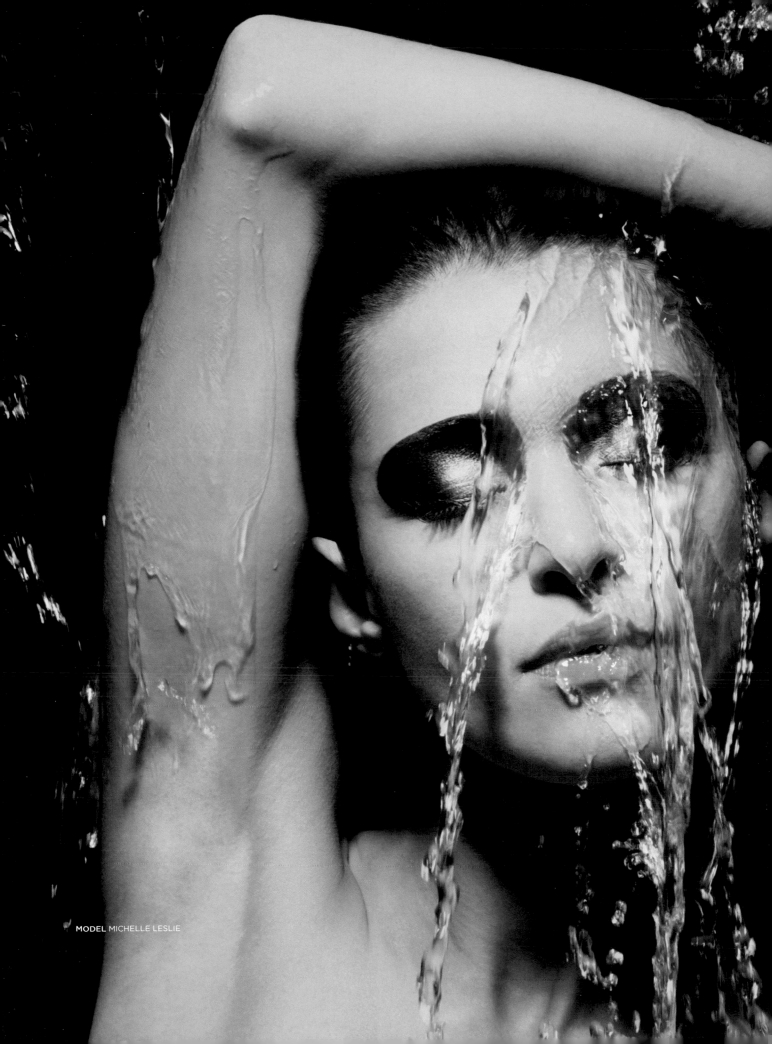

MODEL MICHELLE LESLIE

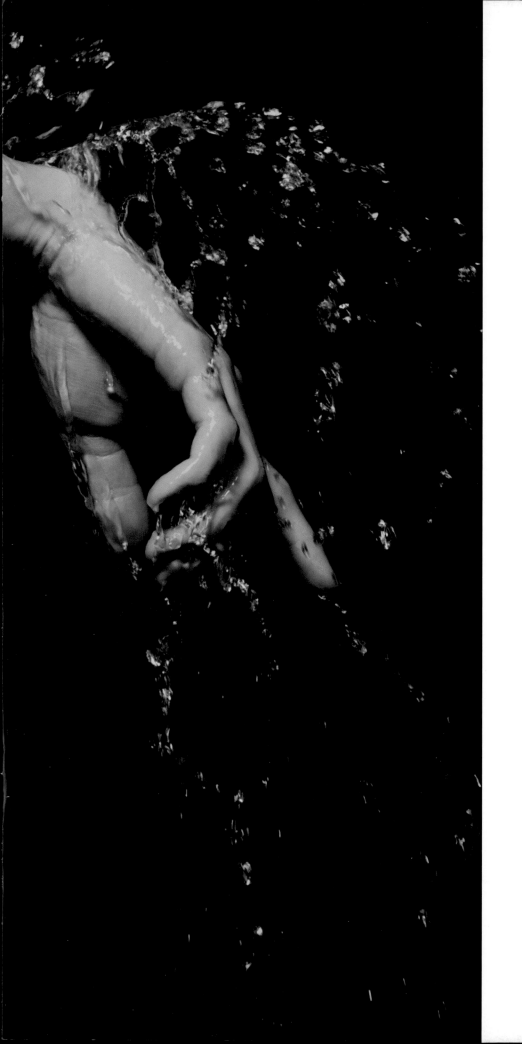

First published in 2012

Copyright © Rae Morris 2012

Copyright © photography Jason Capobianco 2012

Photographs on pages 11 and 16–21 by Steven Chee. Photographs
on pages 12–15 by Katie Nolan.

All rights reserved. No part of this book may be reproduced or
transmitted in any form or by any means, electronic or mechanical,
including photocopying, recording or by any information storage
and retrieval system, without prior permission in writing from
the publisher. The *Australian Copyright Act* 1968 (the Act) allows
a maximum of one chapter or 10 per cent of this book, whichever
is the greater, to be photocopied by any educational institution for
its educational purposes provided that the educational institution
(or body that administers it) has given a remuneration notice to
Copyright Agency Limited (CAL) under the Act.

Arena Books, an imprint of
Allen & Unwin
83 Alexander Street
Crows Nest NSW 2065
Australia
Phone: (61 2) 8425 0100
Fax: (61 2) 9906 2218
Email: info@allenandunwin.com
Web: www.allenandunwin.com

Cataloguing-in-Publication details are available from
the National Library of Australia
www.trove.nla.gov.au

ISBN 978 1 74237 340 9

Design by Stephen Smedley, Tonto Design

Printed in China by Imago

10 9 8 7 6 5 4 3 2 1